FOR YOUR

health

A LOOK INTO GOD'S METHODS FOR HEALING

By Lorna Dueck & Dr. Nell DeBoer

FOR YOUR HEALTH
Copyright © 2018 by Lorna Dueck & Dr. Nell DeBoer

This material is not intended as a substitution for medical advice. Please consult a physician before undertaking any changes to diet, exercise, or medication.

Printed in Canada

ISBN: 978-1-4866-1822-4

Word Alive Press
119 De Baets Street, Winnipeg, MB R2J 3R9
www.wordalivepress.ca

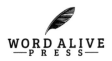
WORD ALIVE
—P R E S S—
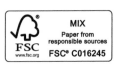
MIX
Paper from
responsible sources
FSC
www.fsc.org
FSC® C016245

Cataloguing in Publication may be obtained through Library and Archives Canada

*To my daughter, and my dear sister-in-law, Margaret.
Your perseverance, suffering, and love exhibited through your
own health challenges have inspired me with a tender heart and
persistence in prayer for healing.*

CONTENTS

ACKNOWLEDGEMENTS

There are more than one hundred people who volunteer to pray for miracles of healing to happen for the 10,000-plus people who phone in each month to the Prayer Lines at 100 Huntley Street/Crossroads Christian Communications.

The faith of these Prayer Partners, the faith of the staff who pray the evening and weekend hours, the staff who lead the technology and responses, and the many real people who have a need for healing that our Prayer Partners daily encounter are a wonder to watch. The faith of these people and their connection to the living Christ has resulted in countless people phoning back to the Prayer Lines to report healing of a wide variety of physical, emotional, and spiritual ailments. Your work in prayer has inspired this book.

A special thank you to Cheryl Weber, Maggie John, and Greg Musselman and their team at 100 Huntley Street who challenge and strengthen me with stories of how God answers the needs of people. For over forty years, the teams at 100 Huntley Street have documented healing stories, and that history of evidence inspired me.

Mike Wright in filming and editing, and Courtney Hinz in story flow and editing, worked hard to compose the collection of interviews in this book that have been gathered for the human experience with healing. Thank you for your art and sensitivity that turned interviewing into a natural story. Thank you to Carla Lowe at Word Alive Press for your careful edit that helped create a book.

Rachelle Melnichuk, my executive assistant, Anson Liske on chase producing, who scoured for details on our stories, thank you for making the scheduling work, protecting the time, screening the stories, and believing this work needed doing.

To Amy Laforet, Barbara Blundell, and Steve Hubley, who design, edit, and produce the final copy of this work for Crossroads, your care and sensitivity has been deeply appreciated.

INTRODUCTION

Healing is hard work. Healing affects every part of body and soul; it plunges from hope to despair; it is the road we hope to never have to travel, but our bodies tell us differently.

I was in my mid-twenties when I was desperate for healing. Migraines crippled me almost daily, and I feared I would lose my job as an administrative clerk because of them. At a noon break, I left my office tower on Portage Avenue in Winnipeg and walked over to St. Mary's Cathedral, relieved to find the door open. I slumped into a pew, pulled down a kneeler, and begged God again for a healing from migraine headaches.

I pleaded, I waited, I bargained that if I could only be migraine-free, I would serve God forever. I returned to my office, but the migraine that day was so bad my husband picked me up; as we drove home, we pulled aside on Pembina Highway so I could throw up. And that has been it for my migraine headaches. I honestly can't recall having a migraine headache in the thirty-plus years that have followed that desperate prayer at St. Mary's.

So perhaps this book is partly payback for that supernatural healing I believe I received, but I do know that if we don't tell the story of healing, we forget it.

I thought of this as I read through an esteemed hospital chaplain's thesis, "Yearning for Wholeness: Interrelationships between Spirituality and Healing." That thesis was the work of Dr. Nell DeBoer, who, for more than thirty years, has cared for the spiritual needs of people in hospital or long-term care on behalf of the Christian Reformed Church. I liked the combination of presence and prayer that Nell brought into health crisis and asked if we could work together on using elements from her thesis for reviving the memory, the truth, and the practice that God is deeply engaged in the physical care of our health needs.

The topic of healing tends to provoke a diverse set of reactions. Some will view it as foundational to their belief, having attended local healing services, rallies boasting famous healers, and perhaps even becoming suspicious of those who don't seem to share the same enthusiasm for the practice that they do. However, others will have grown up in church cultures where healing was an almost "taboo" subject, dismissed as the work of scam artists or fodder for the desperate and gullible. Likely most readers will land somewhere in between. While humble discussions around our theology of healing are certainly important within our church communities, the focus of this book lies elsewhere.

Instead, we begin this writing firmly founded on the biblical belief that God *does* heal. The stories that follow are testimonies of this healing power, and of the diverse methods God uses to bring about these gracious and glorious acts. From what we may initially consider the "medically mundane" to the miraculous, each story is intended to highlight the power and goodness of Jehovah-Rapha, the God Who Heals.

One book simply can't cover all that's needed on healing, and an obvious shortcoming of this volume is that because of time and space, we haven't examined the robust work of healing underway in the Roman Catholic world, limiting ourselves to the tradition we both belong to—Protestant life. We also have not written on the remarkable growth in Christian healing outside of North America, but encourage you to explore those global reports.

Some of you picking up this book may be doing so skeptically, perhaps with a raw and heartbreaking experience at the forefront of your mind in which God did not bring about the healing you prayed so hard for. There is no denying that these situations are mysterious, and often we will never know on this side of eternity why God chose to act one way in one situation, and differently in another. Amid the mystery, the disappointment, and the victories, we must continue to teach in this generation the practice and belief of healing, a renewal of what began with God so many centuries ago.

We hope the following stories illustrate how God can sustain and bring peace even in the midst of suffering, a peace humans cannot conjure up on our own. We have a good and sovereign Shepherd who cared for those society had snubbed, who wept with His friends over the death of their brother (even though He knew in a few moments He would resurrect him), and who Himself bore more pain on the cross than we can ever imagine.

Christ knows suffering, Christ knows our suffering, and Christ is the One who wove our bodies together in the womb and still has the power to untangle any knots that torment us in it today. And we know that whatever should end our days here on earth, whether it be a current illness, an injury, old age many years from now, or the return of Christ the King, this brief collection of moments we have spent here will open into an Eternal Life where brokenness will be forever defeated.

What a Saviour, what a Healer, what a Comforter, what a Friend! It is our prayer that the reminder of Christian history, and the scientific summary of faith's healing effects from Nell's thesis research, will revive your faith in God. It is our hope that the true stories ahead and the experience of people we have met personally in the journey of their healing will bring you hope and turn your hearts to a secure and confident prayer, as well as give you peace in God Almighty, Jehovah-Rapha.

> Jesus went through all the towns and villages, teaching in their synagogues, proclaiming the good news of the kingdom and healing every disease and sickness.
> —MATTHEW 9:35

Chapter 1

A COMMUNITY THAT PRAYED

Though one may be overpowered, two can defend themselves. A cord of three strands is not quickly broken.

—ECCLESIASTES 4:12

Mariette had known trials before. When she was around fifty years old, she was diagnosed with cancer, an illness she would eventually overcome. But increased age and an Alzheimer's diagnosis in 2012 presented a new level of challenge for both Mariette and her family.

"Did I have a body? Did I have a mind? I don't know," says Mariette. "I don't remember anything. I was down to zero."

The first signs of decline occurred when her daughter, Audrey, began getting phone calls from strangers that Mariette had wandered away from her house and had become lost and hungry, unable to find her way home. She started to have transient ischemic attacks (something like small strokes) and her communication skills were clearly deteriorating, sometimes even nonexistent. Audrey knew things could not continue as they were. Mariette would need to be placed somewhere she could receive the increased level of care.

"It's not easy to funnel through information when you're trying to find care for your parent, and it was overwhelming," Audrey admits. She was relieved to find Menno Home, a faith-based care facility in Abbotsford, B.C., for her mother, but describes it as a "devastating experience to leave a loved one behind when you don't understand fully the disease."

Most difficult of all was the feeling Audrey had that she was losing her mother. It seemed Alzheimer's had already stolen Mariette's mind, and Audrey was sure that within the year, Mariette's body would give out, as well. What happened next only furthered Audrey's fears. A short time after arriving in her care home, Mariette suffered a devastating fall from her wheelchair and broke her neck.

At that point, the staff at Mariette's care home didn't think that she would be returning to them. It wasn't her first fall, and the family had become used to hearing that she may not recover with each incident; this time, though, the damage seemed too severe for her to overcome.

"I did not think she would be with us much longer," says Menno Home chaplain, Ingrid Schultz. Chaplain Schultz prayed for healing, and so did others in the community of 700 seniors, Menno Home, where Mariette lived. Ingrid also gently left a prayer shawl on Mariette's shoulders. Shawls are a lovingly knit embrace left on the shoulders of an ailing or lonely resident to remind them they are being prayed for. The shawls are made by residents in independent care, and a normal part of community prayer at Menno Home.

Prayer Shawls and Prayer People
Much to everyone's disbelief, Mariette began to slowly improve. But not only physically; most mysterious and shocking of all was the fact that Mariette began to demonstrate cognitive improvements, as well. While her prior deterioration had made it seem impossible, the improvement of her memory gave Audrey enough hope to try and

encourage other activities for Mariette to exercise her cognitive muscles. She began playing Scrabble with other residents and visitors in her care home. Audrey bought her an iPad and she began playing games that her family members downloaded for her. Ingrid (the chaplain) recruited her to greet and hand out books at chapel services.

Not only was the improvement apparent to her children, friends, and her healthcare staff, but the changes were soon officially documented, as well. Mariette had been given a test to determine whether she was an appropriate fit for the services offered in the care home before she moved in. The test involved thirty questions, of which Mariette could answer five. The next time she was tested, she answered thirteen. In a third test, she answered twenty-one, and in her most recent testing, she answered twenty-nine of the thirty cognitive questions correctly. Mariette now cheerfully volunteers for staff for more than twenty hours a week in the care home where she once lived as a locked-down Alzheimer's patient.

"It was a miraculous change that none of us could even fathom," Ingrid marvels. "It never happens that residents in long-term care improve so much that the doctor and care staff say that they can move to independent living."

"Usually people move from assisted or independent to long-term care, but Mariette came the other way," Ingrid adds.

Mariette is confident she can explain her recovery. "When I look at the people with Alzheimer's and think that I was like that and even much worse, I know there's no way I could have gotten out of that by myself," she says with confidence. "There's no way, without the intervention of God. It had to be God. It's a miracle, because nothing else would have taken me out of there."

"I truly do believe that," Audrey confirms, "because she's my mom again. She's my mom. It's important to have her back."

When asked what she would tell others experiencing what she went through with her mother, Audrey says, "Don't give up. Don't lose hope. Be an advocate for your parent. Find your support system, find your network. There are people out there, there are programs that can help you if you don't understand where to go. They'll navigate through the system for you; they'll help you through."

She continues, "Not knowing that, when it all first happens to you, is scary. It's overwhelming. But there are people in [the care homes] and they have been fantastic with my mother, and they've been fantastic with me, and I'm grateful for that. I can't say enough for the people that I've met through this experience, this journey."

"I feel that prayer is a crucial piece of our work here," says Ingrid, Mariette's care home chaplain. "Not just the chaplains praying, but the residents praying for each other, and other staff in housekeeping, cleaning the room and then coming in and seeing that a resident is in distress or not feeling well or discouraged or grieving and coming in to say a prayer for them. We see this happening every day. It's a community of care, and prayer is at the heart of it."

"There's no word," replies Mariette when she's asked about the role other people have played in her recuperation. "I don't think I know a word strong enough to describe it in English."

"Mariette is a miracle, and she's passing on those prayers and that joy and that compassion onto others. She is a blessing here at Menno Home," says Ingrid. "We're so grateful for her."

Many of us will have the blessing of saying that one of the most beautiful gifts God has given us is our friends and our family. When we get good news at work, when we have a big anniversary, or we reach another big milestone, they're the first ones we call to celebrate with us. By sharing in our joy, they increase it exponentially.

If you've ever been in a situation when you were away from those most important to you and had to celebrate alone, you will know that even the happiest of happenings are somehow quickly drained of their colour when you have no one to share them with.

Grief works in an opposite fashion. Sharing the weight of joy with our friends and family makes it grow; when those whom we love surround us in our times of suffering, their nearness seems to almost parcel out some of the load we're carrying, spreading out the burden and sometimes being the only thing that makes it bearable.

If they functioned in a mathematical sense, companions would be shown to multiply our joy so that our final sum would indicate the initial quantity had increased; conversely, in times of grief, our companions act as divisors, splitting our pain into smaller chunks and leaving our final sum more endurable than when we started.

We read in Ecclesiastes that, *"Though one may be overpowered, two can defend themselves. A cord of three strands is not quickly broken"* (Ecclesiastes 4:12). This verse and our times of joy and grief illustrate a key feature that God has built into humanity: We were *specifically designed* with a need for one another.

"I am just so thankful, there's no word for these things," Mariette answered when asked what it meant to be cared for by her son and daughter. "But the thing is, it's very embarrassing when you realize what they did for you. You can't imagine how much they can do for you. And I can never repay them for that."

Perhaps you've had an experience that makes you able to empathize with Mariette, or maybe you can imagine feeling the same way in her position. Our society values independence, individuality, and the self-made man. But that pride in our self-sufficiency can make things very difficult when we face the inevitable arrival of circumstances in which self no longer proves sufficient.

While hard work and a recognition of one's personal responsibilities is to be commended, the Bible is full of commandments for us to care for one another as a larger community. The New Testament's presentation of the Church as a Body affirms this idea. Your body works as one macro-unit made up of countless micro-units. When you get a cut on your finger, all kinds of cells and organisms rush to the injury to begin the healing process. And so it is when we are suffering.

All three of the women in Mariette's story testified to the instrumental role the community played in their journeys of care or healing. The prayers of the staff and residents at the home, the friends that socialized with Mariette and encouraged her mind to be active, and those who shared their energy and time to help care for her mother when Audrey was growing short on those resources all contributed in critical ways just by their simple, humble obedience, service, and love for Mariette and her daughter.

None of us can manage our journeys alone, nor are we meant to. If we haven't already experienced it, there will come a day when we realize we need help, when we realize all this time that our perception of self-sufficiency was an utter illusion. And though the circumstances that bring us to that place are often difficult, the gifts of humility and acceptance, along with the servant-hearted care from those around us that follows, can sometimes seem to almost make the trial worth it.

Healing can require a community of care. So, let's gather near to those whom we love, thanking God today for the gift He has given us in each other. And let us actively seek to be a practical and spiritual blessing in their lives now, until the day when healing is complete.

Chapter 2

CUT DOWN IN THE PRIME OF LIFE

So God created mankind in his own image, in the image of God he created them; male and female, he
created them.

—GENESIS 1:27

Mathew Embry was only nineteen years old when he received
news that would change his life forever. He was an average
university student, young and active with a full life ahead of him.
But one day, after spending some time outside mountain biking,
Mathew came home and began nonchalantly kicking a ball around
the yard when suddenly he couldn't feel the ball properly with his
foot. Numbness and hypersensitivity spread rapidly from his foot,
and within twenty minutes, it reached all the way up to his chest.
Next, leg spasms and an assortment of other symptoms kicked in. He
was brought to the doctor and before long, he and his family received
the diagnosis: Mathew had Multiple Sclerosis (MS).

The news was a terrible shock. Mathew and his family knew
that the path MS took was unpredictable, but more often than not,
it took a terrible toll on the patient's physical, and occasionally even
mental, capacities—sometimes quite rapidly. The lack of a cure, the

lack of control, and the uncertainty as to what lay ahead led to a state of terror for the whole family.

Unwilling to accept his son's prognosis, Mathew's father, Dr. Ashton Embry, began intense research at the medical library across street where he worked near the University of Calgary. Though Ashton's academic training was in geology, having studied in the field of science at least enabled him to access and study the research around Mathew's new diagnosis in a way that could have been more difficult for someone further removed from the subject.

At the time, there were few treatments available for MS, and those diagnosed weren't given much hope for the future. However, through his research, Mathew's father believed he found evidence that suggested dietary and lifestyle changes may be helpful for managing the disease. The findings required Mathew to cut out dairy, gluten, beans, foods high in sugar, fat, or salt, to decrease the amount of red meat in his diet, as well as increase his intake of fruit vegetables and vitamin D. Finally, Mathew had to ensure he was getting an appropriate amount of exercise. But the threat of the illness and the desperation for a cure motivated Mathew to maintain his new habits with his family's support.

The initial fear and desperation brought on by Mathew's diagnosis had caused his father to move quite quickly in his research, and by the time Mathew went to his first appointment at the MS clinic, he had already started his strict new health regimen. When the neurologist came in and casually suggested Mathew and his dad grab a donut and coffee while they waited for their appointment, Ashton couldn't help but let out an incredulous laugh. It didn't take long for the father and son to realize that the two of them didn't see eye-to-eye with the MS clinic when it came to determining the best route for managing Mathew's illness. They decided to forego the clinic's treatment and to stick to their own diet- and exercise-based approach instead.

Mathew received his diagnosis in 1995, and by all appearances, his disciplined approach to his health has paid off. Though maintaining such a strict regimen hasn't always been easy, today, Mathew is still active and independent, and lives a life much like any other man his age, despite receiving his MS diagnosis more than twenty years ago.

In the past several years, Matt has created an advocacy group, MS HOPE, as well as the award-winning documentary, "Living Proof," to give others who have been diagnosed with MS evidence that there are steps they can take to actively manage their disease.

"Sometimes I tell people to see food as a drug," Mathew says. "When you wake up in the morning, one of the first decisions you make when you're having breakfast is what you're going to put in your mouth.

"Well, then that continues throughout the day," he goes on. "So you have three meals a day, you may have snacks, and each time you're eating, if you read the science and realize how important diet is for these conditions, you start to see you're taking control back."

Yet More To Be Healed

After his dive into healing for MS, there were still two significant symptoms that plagued Mathew: depression and anxiety.

"You know, I was raised in a very scientific-minded household with very limited exposure to the church. And I think that scientific rigour, and that approach we had, was instrumental in learning about, say, the dietary therapies, and the exercise that helped me regain my health. And it was those scientific principles that really applied to life," says Mathew.

This was for Mathew's physical healing, but anxiety, alcoholism, depression, and a life of telling lies to get where he needed to go pushed Mathew beyond physical healing.

"It was truth that I first committed my life to," he shares. "Then it was Jesus Christ after that. Once I realized that Jesus Christ said He was the truth—if that makes sense, it's hard to explain—but once I recognized that truth was the key to life, I worked to tell the most truth I could possibly tell on a day-to-day basis. And then, through that, once I understood that Jesus was the truth, well, then I had to learn the way," says Mathew.

"And that was a whole other step," he continues. "I'm still growing in that. And trying to understand that. When I accepted Jesus Christ and started to live in Jesus Christ, I watched both those issues of anxiety and depression disappear."

Mathew is my colleague, an outstanding Executive Producer at YES TV working from our Calgary office. Those of us who have the joy of working with Mathew find his beliefs as a Christian not only inspiring to our physical health, but also instructive to our spiritual health. Mathew is regimented about everything he eats, and his exercise routine—even when on the road or enjoying hospitality in our homes.

"When we control and we're really disciplined about our exercise and how we eat, it's also a form of spiritual discipline," explains Mathew. "There is this one layer in the physical world which we live in, [physical] healing, and you're seeing those transformations happen, but on a very deep level, I think it's also about spiritual discipline and obedience.

"That motivation is stronger the more I work with God," he goes on. "The more I pray, the more I'm thankful, the more I'm grateful, and the more that I see that all interactions are from God and an opportunity for me to act in Christ, then I get stronger."

Mathew continues to be an advocate for our best physical health, and I can't help but wonder if his unique path to faith in Christ, his father's scientific approach to food as medicine, and Mathew's own driving force have all been part of God's method for healing Mathew of his MS symptoms. He sits in a unique position from which to coach people in healing.

"Feeling hopeless and helpless is really to me about feeling a lack of control. And the problem with these illnesses and with all illness is fear, and fear comes from an uncontrollable future. My advice to people is the best way to get rid of that fear is to act in the now," says Mathew. "To think about, okay, the future is purely an illusion. You are conjuring up images in your mind, and for most people those are scary, horrible images. Well, it's not real.

"So, try your best to focus on reality," he encourages. "What's right in front of you, the next right decision that you can make. Whether that be your diet, exercise, how you treat people, forgiveness, being thankful, being grateful. Whatever that next decision is now, try to make the best one. And God will give you the opportunity to make the right choice if you do it.

"So whether it be diet, make the right choice. Whether it be exercise, you know, why not? Whether it be treating someone or forgiving someone in the past, whatever the case, whatever you can do in the now to make your life good, try it.

"This may sound bizarre," Mathew continues, "but I sometimes see MS HOPE as a training ground. That God gave me this disease and this suffering for me to understand what it's like to suffer. And how to stand up to give people hope. Well, that's through MS and one story. Now my next mission is to share the story of Jesus Christ. Because there are a lot of people who need that hope and who are suffering from other conditions that Christ can heal."

Chapter 3

SHOULD I TRUST A FAITH HEALER?

Is anyone among you sick? Let them call the elders of
the church to pray over them and anoint them with oil
in the name of the Lord.
—JAMES 5:14

People employed as clergy should have a leading edge on the practice and understanding of healing. This chapter takes a bit more space to examine three powerful people operating in the work of pastoral care and healing.

"It Was Like a Light Switch Went Off..."
Healing was never a major part of Paul Teske's faith experience growing up or at his Lutheran seminary, or while serving as a Navy chaplain for twenty-two years. While Paul vaguely believed healing was still possible, it seemed more like something that just happened for Jesus and His apostles in the Early Church.

However, after having experienced the Holy Spirit's working in some incredible ways, Paul began studying New Testament passages on healing and became convicted that he was biblically mandated to seek healing for the sick. He began praying for church members, and through following the instructions of James 5:14, he saw four people healed over a ten-year period. It was at this point that Paul was speaking at a conference when he suffered a sudden cerebral hemorrhage.

"It was like a light switch went off. One minute I could shift my weight and the next minute I was completely paralyzed on my left side," Paul recalls. "[It was a] very sobering moment...and confusing."

Paul was hospitalized for two weeks. But during that period, he felt God telling him through a passage in Hosea that he was going to be healed. And soon, in fact, Paul was convinced God wanted to heal him within twenty-one days of his stroke, a healing that, if delivered by "deadline," would have to occur on May 28, 2004.

Paul had known a woman in his church who had been healed of Stage Four breast cancer at a healing service and he believed he could also find hope at such an event. So, just twenty-one days after his stroke, Paul's wife drove him to a service with faith healer Benny Hinn. Under the direction of an usher, Paul seated himself in the front row without his walker, which the usher had taken to the side. Two and a half hours into the four-hour service, Paul experienced healing during the music and worship. Miraculously, it was May 28, 2004.

Paul and his wife were suddenly called to the front by Rev. Hinn; surprisingly, Paul used his regained ability to walk independently to approach the evangelist. Benny Hinn went on to declare to Paul that God had healed him, and when he had, Benny told Paul that he believed God was now going to use Paul to heal the people back home in his Lutheran congregation in Connecticut. Paul went home and that Sunday, prayed for and witnessed two people experience healing in his church. He believed the message Benny Hinn had given him was true.

In the years since, Paul has been faithful to that conviction that God calls us to pray and seek healing for one another. In doing so, he has had the privilege of seeing countless people healed and has testified to the goodness of God and His gospel message to all those for whom he prays.[1]

"This Is Kind of Crazy..."

The day Reverend Robbie Dawkins believed he was called to the work of healing happened unexpectedly. He received a phone call asking for healing, but he was in a bad mood, angry with his senior pastor and not feeling in a good place to minister to someone. Yet the woman on the other end of the line was desperate; her father was going in for open-heart surgery and the prognosis was not good.

Robbie remembers the call clearly. "They weren't believers, and so she just called the church and literally said, 'Rub some beads or burn the candle. I don't know what you people do, but I just need somebody to do *something*.' And so, I said I could pray."

Robbie speaks of his attitude as he started. "I was just praying, you know, 'Lord just be with them in this time of loss; comfort them.' There was no prayer for healing—everybody I'd prayed for before died or got worse. And so, I had no expectation that anything would happen.

"But then I just heard the Lord say, 'Get out on a limb.' And I didn't even know what that meant. And then I heard Him say in my spirit, not in an audible voice but in my spirit, said, 'Open your mouth and I'll fill it.'"

Almost to his own surprise, Robbie suddenly prayed that the man would receive a new heart. Not only that, he told the woman that God was going to heal her father's lungs, as well, something she hadn't even mentioned.

"And as I heard myself say it, I started panicking," Robbie remembers. "I started telling her, 'I'm no healer, I've never seen healing—everybody I've prayed for gets worse.'" Robbie went on desperately backtracking, but the woman just incredulously repeated what he had prayed for and hung up.

Robbie couldn't believe what he had done and was worried about what the consequences of his actions would be. "I thought it was like an exposé show with somebody trying to catch preachers who promised healing but couldn't deliver." But his fears were soon completely turned around.

The woman called back an hour and a half later. God had answered the prayer he had placed in Robbie's mouth. The man's heart showed no signs of the two previous bypass surgeries he had received, and his lungs were fully restored, as well. Robbie couldn't believe the woman crying and sobbing at the other end of the line and still didn't until he saw documentation from the hospital for himself.

This experience completely changed Robbie's perspective. He reports he has since prayed for and witnessed countless awe-inspiring acts of God's healing and now believes healing is something the church is called to fight for.

"We can use the authority He's given us to step out and see the sick healed," Robbie says with confidence, "God doesn't tell me specifically to pray for each person I pray for, but the Scriptures say heal the sick, raise the dead, etc., so with each of those situations, we just step into it because we have the authority to do that."

Robbie's confidence in God's power and His compassion for the suffering drive him on, keeping him praying for healing and life here on earth until the day when *There will be no more death or mourning or crying or pain, for the old order of things has passed away*" (Revelation 21:4).[2]

Faith healers are certainly controversial, but my policy is to unpack their actions and teachings and examine what is at work. I evaluate faith healers "by their fruits," following the warning Jesus gave in

Matthew 7:15–20 for sorting out the false prophets He told us would come along. Jesus asked, *"By their fruit you will recognize them. Do people pick grapes from thornbushes, or figs from thistles? Likewise, every good tree bears good fruit, but a bad tree bears bad fruit"* (Matthew 7:16–17).

We've chosen to explore clergy who are reputed as faith healers, Paul Teske and Robbie Dawkins, because they are good "fruit" people.

To some degree, skepticism is healthy and reasonable. But as Christians, the anchor of our hope, Jesus, is fully man, but He is also fully God. The God whom in the earliest record of walking with the human race declared in Exodus 15:26, *"...I am the Lord, who heals you."* This is the God who does not sleep, but who has watched over you every night of your life while you do (Psalm 121). The God who always acts in love, and who never acts in malice, selfishness, manipulation, or wickedness, the Perfect Father, the Good Shepherd, the Wonderful Counselor, the Comforter, and our Friend.

When we pray for healing, this is the to whom God we are praying. Why should we be at all surprised, then, when we hear miraculous stories of restoration?

"You know, people ask me all the time why God won't heal everybody. I say I don't know, I don't know," says Paul. "I preach the gospel every Sunday and not everybody is saved; sometimes nobody is saved. But I don't quit preaching. I pray for the sick all the time; some are healed, some aren't. I don't quit praying for people because they're not all healed. That would be ludicrous. What I've learnt about God is that, in all this, whether it's teaching or preaching or healing, He's good, and I can trust Him, and He knows what He's doing. So if you are healed and somebody else isn't, that's God's choice. I'm just praying. My job is to pray."

Paul continues, "You know, I was telling somebody a while ago, Moses' job was to raise the stick, God had the hard part to split the

16

waters. My job is to raise the stick, God's job is to part the waters. So, if you ask me to raise the stick, I'm going to do it. And we'll see what God's gonna do."

Perhaps hearing things like this frighten us. If we can't be sure that God will bring healing a hundred percent of the time, how can we fully place our trust in Him? The reason that we can is because we don't trust in God for healing only; we trust in Him for so much more.

"We have to remember the resurrection. If there's no resurrection, I'm in the wrong business," Paul says. "We're all eventually going to die. But death is simply the threshold into eternal life, where we are going live forever. No more pain, no more sorrow, no more suffering, all joy. So we can't lose sight of that. You know death is not the end; it's the beginning."

Are There Some Special Words to Pray?

Robbie Dawkins has travelled to many churches who carry the teachings of the Pentecostal tradition and he has worked worldwide in healing ministry. Both Dawkins and his followers are brimming with evidence and anecdotes of healings, but because of time and distance, it was difficult for me to track the accuracy of those claims.

What I do know for a fact is the good fruit of Dawkins' humble service of showing up where needed for healing. Robbie is also important to study because of his widespread appeal among young, charismatic believers. I caught up with Robbie Dawkins for an in-person teaching at a small Vineyard church plant in downtown Toronto during summer 2018. I asked Robbie if there were specific words needed for a healing.

"I don't think there are specific words, necessarily, but Jesus is pretty consistent; be healed, rise up and walk, stretch out your hand—there has to be words of command," says Dawkins. "This body comes from the earth, it was formed from the earth, this physical being. And when we command the body, we are taking dominion over the earth, because it comes from the earth and we are commanding it.

"So if I pray for your shoulder, I'm not commanding you to do anything, I'm commanding this body that comes from the earth, that God gave human beings dominion over, rule over, to come into alignment with God's plan and purpose that he originally had. And so, when we command the body, asking the Lord to come and heal somebody is like asking your boss to come and do your job for you."

I then asked Robbie if he had everything in his own physical body healed that needed healing.

"No! No!" he shakes his head. "My knees, I'm contending for healing in my knees. I have bad thyroids that went bad about twenty-five years ago. I've prayed for and seen four different people get brand-new thyroids and I'm still contending for mine, my knees contending for them to be healed and you know, it's war, we are engaging in war."

While writing this book, I reflected on four male friends of mine who were hit hard by cancer in the past twelve months. Jim Olson was just three weeks from diagnosis to death with anaplastic thyroid cancer, despite having a formidable tribe of righteous people praying fervently for his healing and the best of medical care. I still don't understand that loss.

Trust in a Heavenly Healing

Another friend, Dr. Lon Allison, has had a little more time to teach on the lessons of living with a fatal disease. After forty-seven years of being a minister of the gospel, after three supernatural healings of smaller ailments in his own body, Lon lived a life of rigorous discipline in exercise and spiritual activity.

A healthy, symptom-free Lon received unusual bloodwork back from a routine physical in 2017 when he was age sixty-five. "It would be cancer, the awful, awful kind, the worst of all possible liver cancers;

intrahepatic cholangiocarcinoma," Lon shares. As he visits with me, he says, "I'm at absolute peace because of the guarantee of my healing... Apart from God's superintending for this world, I am going to be healed in heaven. What's helped me be at peace—spiritually, I have an absolute trust in the sovereignty of God. The two doctrines sustain me: the sovereignty of God—nothing happens apart from his awareness—and secondly, the love of God. These are the two foundations of my peace of where and when my healing will be done."

In his much-loved work as minister of the gospel, Lon says he has prayed for hundreds of people to be healed, and many have been. As past Director of the Billy Graham Center, having pastored several churches, people care deeply for Lon, his wife Marie, and their children.

"People have come crying at my door feeling called to pray for my physical healing. It's a Monday morning, 8:00 a.m., a guy knocked on my door. 'God has told me to heal you. God has told me you are going to be healed.' So he laid his hands on me and I am 'Amen-ing' the whole way through, and then it didn't happen immediately, or next week, or next month and honestly, I haven't seen that guy in church in a long time," says Lon.

"Healing isn't even a question for me, it's only a matter of where and when. Did we search out therapies, both medical and holistic? Yes, but not in lieu of the spiritual search," he continues. "I spent more time meditating on the sovereignty and love of God than I did on thinking of chemotherapy vs radiation and so on. The benefit is that it gave us a spiritual buoyancy through everything. Marie and I have felt in a bubble of grace.

"I've been amazed at how singularly focused Christians are on being healed in this world," he adds. "It's at the level of idolatry in the western world, that how can anyone want to go to heaven right now? Wow, we've made too much of these seventy years."

In what could be the last year of his life, Lon is still all about the work of teaching the gospel, travelling for evangelism, and mentoring others. I'm one who has been in Lon's leadership group for sixteen years, and doubted that in a year of fatal cancer, he should spend the annual four-day retreat away from his family. He scoffed at my own protectionism of my now-grown family, challenging me to place Christ first.

"The inner life healing that Marie and I have enjoyed through this I never would have expected," says Lon. "The highs are higher, and the lows are more meaningful lows. As a pastor, I absolutely believe that when someone is ill or diseased that when I lay hands on them and pray, that God can [and may] heal their body. And if God only heals one out of one hundred, no wonder we quit believing.

"But I always believe God answers the prayer that the inner soul of the person can be rich and at peace if they believe. If someone is consumed by their disease, consumed about getting well, then I think they are probably in sin because they have made health an idol. I have never seen the righteous not have peace in the face of terminal illness. I think the Holy Spirit wants to heal people's hearts; I've never seen the righteous ones who are suffering greatly not have the optimistic glow of God's presence and control."

Lon has spent plenty of work in the quiet place of his Bible, prayer and journaling, and with Christian friends, developing his life into that which I would describe as a "righteous one."

As this book went to print, I received a note from Lon, celebrating that his cancer has gone into partial remission. "It is declining, though still present," he shares. "My energy and vigour remain high, my liver is operating at one hundred percent. It doesn't mean cancer-free, but we'll take partial remission and be thankful."

In keeping with the mystery that is our God, our next story is another righteous friend who was healed on earth from a fatal cancer diagnosis.

Chapter 4

THE DOCTOR
NEEDS A DOCTOR

Praise the Lord, my soul; all my inmost being, praise
his holy name. Praise the Lord, my soul, and forget not
all his benefits—who forgives all your sins and heals
all your diseases, who redeems your life from the pit
and crowns you with love and compassion, who satis-
fies your desires with good things so that your youth
is renewed like the eagle's.
—PSALM 103:1–5

D r. Chuck Borsellino was busy in his clinical practice of neuro-
psychology doing rounds of thirteen patients a day, and somewhere in the routine he noticed a small lump underneath the left side
of his jaw. He thought it should probably be seen by another doctor.
For a few months, his primary care physician thought it was just a
swollen lymph node. But when it didn't seem to go away, she referred
him for a biopsy for more information.

"I remember it was a Friday afternoon," Chuck recalls. "We went
in for a biopsy, and they came back right away. They said, 'We have
some bad news for you. This is cancerous.'"

Chuck continues, "To phone your kids, each one, and to say, 'Dad's got cancer' is a tough, tough phone call to make. And to hear their voice crack, and to know that their life just changed because my life just changed. It was hard for me to see that happen."

Chuck and his wife Jenni were sent to the oncology department at a nearby hospital. Amid their fears, they felt some optimism in the fact that it was known to be a particularly good hospital for treating cancer. However, upon arrival, their hopes quickly turned to disappointment.

"They said, 'We don't accept your insurance.' And we said, 'All right, that's okay, we'll phone the ENT (ear, nose, and throat) specialist, and get another referral to somebody else.' The woman said, 'You don't understand; this is the only place that you can go for what you have.' We asked her what we were supposed to do, and she said, 'I don't know. But here is your only option.'"

Chuck and his wife went home, got down on their knees in their study, and prayed. "We said, 'God, we need a miracle. We need a miracle. We don't know how that's going to happen, but we need a miracle.' And the next morning at 8:00 a.m., the phone rings, 'Hi, this is UT Southwestern trying to set up your appointment.' 'What?' I said back, 'I thought our insurance didn't—' 'Oh that's all taken care of,' the woman said. 'Don't worry about it. It's taken care of.'"

Chuck and his wife still don't understand what had happened that day to change their circumstances, but they knew there was still a long road ahead of them. They went to the appointment to get a better idea of Chuck's prognosis.

"They took a look at several scans and several biopsies, and they said, 'We have some very bad news for you. You have stage four metastatic squamous carcinoma. Which means it's the worst form and its already travelled. It started at the base of your tongue, it's gone under your throat, it's in your lymph nodes, and it's in your lungs. And because it's metastasized so far, there's nothing we can do.'"

Chuck remembers hearing the news. "Your world changes at that moment," he says. "I looked over at Jenni, and I remember her just thinking and saying, 'No, no, no.' And I thought, 'Okay, if it's time for me to die, it's time for me to die. But the helplessness that you feel—to not be able to fix things for your wife and for your kids is a real struggle. So that was the worst time, and we lived with that for probably two weeks."

"Honestly, for a while I felt so numb, I didn't feel God's presence. Not that He wasn't there, but I think that there was a numbness that I felt that made it very difficult for me to sense God's presence. And I remember thinking, 'Well God, at this time of my life, where are you? Where are you?' And then I read Romans 8:34–39 and believed He was saying, 'I am interceding for you. That's where I am; I am interceding for you.'"

Bolted Down for Healing

Chuck went in for more appointments. And in the course of doing so, his diagnosis changed. The doctors realized the cancer was different from what they had originally thought, and that treatment was an option after all.

Chuck recalls, "They told me, 'You're going to have forty-eight radiation treatments, eight chemotherapy treatments, and that's the beginning, that's where we're going to start. We're going to hit you with everything we've got because we only have one shot at this.'"

The radiation treatments, with Chuck bolted down under a plastic mold of his head, neck, and shoulders, were very uncomfortable. "On the treatment table, I became a little bit claustrophobic, and I would pray. 'Dear God, be with me. Help me. I trust you.' And I would sing to myself a worship chorus for the next twenty minutes, and then they would come in and say, 'Okay, it's done, you're done for today,'" says Chuck.

The side-effects were unpleasant, as well. The loss of the ability to swallow, a feeding tube that resulted in a loss of fifty-five pounds, and fried taste buds and salivary glands made even everyday functions that many of us take for granted difficult, but Chuck and his family carried on.

Once Chuck completed his scheduled treatments, the doctors performed a surgery to tighten up the muscles in his neck; three months later, they did another scan and felt one more surgery was necessary to remove the last remaining cancerous spot.

Thinking the surgery would last about an hour, the doctors weren't concerned about its success, and comforted the family that they didn't have much to worry about. However, four-and-a-half hours later, things had clearly gone differently from what they had expected.

"They saw that the cancer had affected the sternocleidomastoid muscle, which is the big muscle in your neck, the lymph nodes, and even the jugular vein, so they took all that out," Chuck explains, "So then it was probably a couple of weeks of recovering from that surgery on my neck, and a little physical therapy to try to get back. This side of my head is numb, and my arm I can't lift above a certain height.

"But that's okay," he continues. "The lesson is that I focus on the life that's left, not what's lost. And that for me, gives me hope for where I'm going. God's given me more days, so I want to use those for His kingdom."

Pursuing Another Round of Prayer

In the early weeks following surgery, Chuck and his wife took the referral of a friend to attend a faith healing service in their Texas city.

"We walk in, we listen to him speak, and then he says, 'If you want prayer, come forward.' Before we could move, probably 100 to 150 people move forward for prayer. You couldn't even get close to the altar! So I thought, 'Oh boy. Now what do I do?' And I thought,

'I'm not coming this far, we're not coming this far to go out the back door. We're gonna get prayed for,'" says Chuck.

"Finally, the preacher said, 'If you've been prayed for, leave room for others,' which gave us a chance to move forward. So we move forward, he comes close to us and I can hear Jenni saying, 'He has cancer, my husband has cancer, he has cancer.' And [he lays] his hands on me and [prays] for me, and I—nothing, I didn't feel any different. So we stayed at the altar to pray.

"And about ten or fifteen minutes later, somebody comes over and says, 'I was on the other side of the altar; God told me to come pray for you.' And then he says, 'I don't know anything about your life or what's going on, but God told me this,' and he put his hand on my head, and he said, 'He's adding years to your life, he's adding years to your life, God's adding years to your life, years to your life.' And I accept that. God's adding years to my life to do one more thing for the kingdom," recalls Chuck.

While still in a season of health monitoring during my interview with him, Chuck has no signs of returned cancer. "I think God uses many ways to touch a life. He uses physicians, and psychologists and physical therapists and so on to perform a miracle in somebody's life. Other times, God heals us instantly," says Chuck. "I had a number of people praying for me, and I think that had an effect—I know that had an effect. I don't understand that exactly, but I believe prayer changes things and all those people who prayed for me made a significant difference in my recovery."

For most of us who experience recovery from a health issue, the medical system will play some role. Whether the doctors themselves believe it or not, they are creations under God's sovereignty who have been granted their knowledge, skills, opportunities, and experience by their Maker. Under His common grace, He has delegated gifts and knowledge and talents to each one of us, with the intention that we would bless and serve one another. This is an expression of goodness and love not only to the receiver of the gift, but also to those who will need those gifts.

Yet when we're sitting in a hospital with cold white walls, strange smells, and scary pamphlet displays hung on the walls, it can be hard to remember it's a place that is teeming with the fingerprints of God. God isn't frightened of such a place, nor is He frightened of the illnesses and fears its walls contain. This is the God who already stormed the gates of hell and defeated death.

Whether or not you feel it, God is present; He is watching over you, and He is overseeing and directing the care you receive. Sometimes, your doctors will get to witness a miracle from the hand of God, and other times, the doctor might be the miracle from the hand of God. There's no reason to be any less thankful or in awe of God in the second case.

Luke 17: 10–19 contains the story of how Jesus comes across ten outcasts exiled from their communities due to the contagious skin infection of leprosy. The men beg for Jesus to heal them, and Jesus immediately grants their request. Overjoyed, the men dance and leap for joy, running off to celebrate their freshly restored physical and social states with their families and communities.

In light of all the excitement, only one man comes back to thank Jesus for His (somewhat major) role in the restoration. The others are far too relieved and eager to rush back into everything they've been missing to remember the One who made such a return possible.

When the story involves a direct and instantaneous miracle from a physically present Jesus Christ, it can feel hard to relate to the re-actions of the people who experienced it. But what if we think about cases of more subtle miracles? Of extensive radiation treatment heal-ing, or a long road to recovery; would we have the same trouble relat-ing to ungratefulness then?

When we experience healing in more "conventional" ways, it may be harder to remember to be thankful. We may subconsciously (or even openly) credit mainly the doctors or our treatment for our healing, forgetting entirely that God was behind those doctors, researchers, and pharmacologists, giving them life and bringing them into the world, then later giving them the ability to create and carry out the treatment that brought you healing. God is the One who originally created your body and all its incredible defense mechanisms that help it fight to restore itself to health, and He's the One who sustains and goads those mechanisms on in your illness. When you think about it, "conventional" doesn't seem like quite the appropriate word for that kind of healing, does it?

However our healing may come about, remember God's hand has accomplished it. Whether He invites some of the people He created into the process or whether He brings it about instantaneously and without their involvement, let's always remember to return to our Saviour, thanking and praising Him for both the current and the eternal restoration He has brought us.

Dr. Chuck Borsellino thinks that hope is there for all who need a healing. "And I pray that you bend a knee and say, 'God, I need you, I need you.' And watch what God can do. Because he can do things that others cannot. Oh, your insurance? It's taken care of. I don't understand that. Still don't understand that. But God took care of it in ways that man couldn't," says Chuck.

"And I just encourage you, to call on God. Jehovah-Rapha, the God that heals. To wipe a tear, to mend a heartache. To deal with a loss, and give you life beyond your loss. That's what I pray for you."

"Praise the Lord, my soul...who forgives all your sins and heals all your diseases" (Psalm 103:1–3).

Chapter 5

WHAT DOES THE BIBLE SAY ABOUT HEALING?

For everything that was written in the past was written to teach us, so that through the endurance taught
in the Scriptures and the encouragement they provide we might have hope.
—ROMANS 15:4

In order to understand the healing practices to which we are called,
it's important to go back to the Scriptures, to look at them in light
of the context in which they occurred, and in reference to the Bible
as a whole. We also want to refer to church history to trace how
healing theology has been interpreted through the ages, and to understand how particularly weighty interpretations have influenced
our views today.

The general tone regarding healing in the Old Testament was
very much one of health and wellbeing as a consequence of individual and national faithfulness to God and God's laws. When the way of
life of God's people was consistent with God's intentions in all areas of
life, the result was greater wholeness and wellbeing.

We read in Exodus 15:25b and 26 that after Moses had led the Israelites out of Egypt into the wilderness, God gave them laws and put them to the test. God said to them:

> If you listen carefully to the Lord your God and do what is right in his eyes, if you pay attention to his commands and keep all his decrees, I will not bring on you any of the diseases I brought on the Egyptians, for I am the Lord, who heals you.
>
> —EXODUS 15:26

The God Who Wounds and Heals

Deuteronomy 32:39 sums up the basic tone of much of the Old Testament: *"See now that I myself am he! There is no god besides me. I put to death and I bring to life, I have wounded and I will heal, and no one can deliver out of my hand."*

This is quite in keeping with what God had said earlier to Moses in Exodus 4:11: *"Who gave human beings their mouths? Who makes them deaf or mute? Who gives them sight or makes them blind? Is it not I, the Lord?"* God was generally understood to be the giver of good as well as of evil. Numerous Scripture passages attest to this understanding.

For the ancient Israelites, there was no question that God could heal and, indeed, was their Healer. Children were given to women who were barren, among them Sarah, the mother of Isaac, when she was well past child-bearing age,[3] and the Shunammite woman.[4] Counted among the stories of healing are Elijah and Elisha healing a child,[5] Elisha cleansing Naaman's leprosy;[6] even a man was raised from the dead when his dead body touched the bones of Elisha.[7]

However, in the Old Testament, God was also seen as being responsible for misfortune and illness. These were recognized as God's

29

chastisement for sin, with a view to helping individuals and the nation of Israel turn to their God. This view, however, is not the only one we find in the Old Testament.

Job, a righteous man who was richly blessed by God, quite unexpectedly lost everything and was overwhelmed with suffering. Because of their view of sickness and disaster as a consequence of sin, Job was ridiculed by family, neighbours, and friends, ending up on the village dump, scratching his sores with shards of pottery. Job challenged their understanding and maintained his innocence, declaring that he had always walked in the ways of God.

In the end, God justified, healed, and restored Job and blessed him with abundantly more than he ever had before. Author Morton Kelsey, theologian, Episcopal priest, and psychologist, notes that no reason was ultimately given for his suffering, though his friends were rebuked because their "inflexible application of this theology had become a religious straitjacket, leading them to speak incorrectly about the Lord's dealing with his servant in this particular case."[8]

The overall tone of the Old Testament, expressed in a number of Psalms, particularly Psalm 103, is that God forgives all our iniquities, and heals all our diseases, and is merciful and gracious, slow to anger and abounding in steadfast love to all who worship and serve Him.

The Healing Ministry of Jesus

Kelsey suggests that this more subtle and gracious strand of Old Testament belief, as reflected in Psalm 103, was at the heart of the healing ministry of Jesus and was further developed in the New Testament.[9] Beate Jakob, a German doctor and theologian who specializes in the role of the church in health, suggests that "understanding Jesus' healing miracles is essential to interpreting Jesus' healing ministry."[10] Jakob reflects that:

Jesus' healing miracles must be interpreted within the framework of the Kingdom of God. These miracles do not primarily present Jesus as a miraculous healer to be consulted in case of disease. Rather, they show that through Jesus, God devotes God's attention to this world completely and forever.[11]

Healing must be seen as a part of the salvation that Jesus came to bring. Together, salvation and healing mark the starting point of a new creation that was already promised in the Old Testament. Jakob comments that:

Jesus' miracles...are not his identity card, but they are signs or signals of God's Kingdom. Jesus' healings do not primarily provide physical or psychological health to individuals but rather provide an invitation for people to come into contact with God.[12]

In Mark 1:35–38, we read that Jesus often withdrew when people wanted to see Him perform miracles or discouraged those who had been healed from proclaiming it, as in Mark 1:43–44. Jakob suggests this is because "Jesus does not want the healing to be misunderstood and separated from the framework of his Gospel."[13]

Jesus' ministry of compassion and healing often put him at odds with the Jewish religious leaders, especially when Jesus challenged their laws and interpretations and healed on the Sabbath. It's not surprising that Jesus did not heal many of them. They weren't open to either Jesus' healings or message of the coming of God's reign among them, and didn't consider either as having come from God.

The ministry of Jesus was one of preaching and healing. This is the model Jesus passed on to His disciples. On at least two occasions during His earthly ministry, He sent them out to do exactly that.

In Matthew 10:7–8, we read that Jesus sent out the twelve with instructions to go and proclaim the Good News, for "the kingdom of heaven has come near." They were to cure the sick, raise the dead, cleanse the lepers, and cast out demons. In Luke 10:9, Jesus' instructions to the seventy sent out in pairs included curing the sick, and telling them, "The kingdom of God has come near to you." Many people came to faith and were healed as a result of the disciples' ministry.

The Healing Ministry of the Apostles

It's not until after the outpouring of the Holy Spirit at Pentecost that we find the disciples, now apostles, continuing with Jesus' ministry. We observed that, while Jesus was still on earth, He had sent His disciples out on two occasions to practice what they had witnessed Jesus doing, that is, preaching and healing.

Following his resurrection, Jesus had instructed the disciples to wait in Jerusalem for the outpouring of the Holy Spirit after He had returned to God. Once empowered by the Holy Spirit, they were to go out into the world to carry on His ministry of proclaiming the Good News of God's salvation and healing the sick. We know from The Acts of the Apostles that they were faithful to Jesus' instructions and their ministry was richly blessed.

The disciples were all together when the Holy Spirit was poured out upon them, enabling them to speak in different languages. Peter (it seems immediately and certainly unabashedly) proclaimed publicly and eloquently, to all who gathered, the Good News of God's coming among humanity in the person of Jesus Christ.[14] There were many visitors in Jerusalem for the Jewish Holy Days and they were amazed and astonished to hear the apostles speaking to them, each in their own language, about God's deeds of power.

Soon after many of the listeners had accepted the message of the God's salvation, the first miracle of the apostles was recorded. Peter and John were going to the temple to pray. Sitting outside the gate was a man, lame from birth, begging for alms. Peter reached out his hand to the man and lifted him up. Immediately, his feet and ankles were made strong and he began walking, leaping, and praising God for his amazing recovery. As a crowd gathered, Peter again took advantage of the opportunity to preach the gospel of Jesus. The apostles were quick to point out that it was not by their own power or piety that this man was healed; rather, it was through faith in Jesus Christ, whom God had sent among them.[15]

When Healing Didn't Come

The apostles appear to have been able to heal, through the power of Jesus, those who were placed on their path in the context of their ministry. Yet there are four notable exceptions when healing does not appear to have been readily given to those suffering from physical illness.[16]

Perhaps the most notable of these instances is that of Paul himself who prayed on three occasions for the removal of "a thorn in the flesh."[17] God's response to him was: *"My grace is sufficient for you, for my power is made perfect in weakness"* (2 Corinthians 12:9). Paul's interpretation was that God did not remove this "thorn" in order to help him stay humble and dependent upon God in all circumstances.

Others, whose illnesses do not appear to have been healed miraculously, were close associates of Paul. Epaphroditus was a leader of the Church of Philippi, and brought gifts from that Christian community to encourage and help Paul in prison in Rome. While there, Epaphroditus contracted an acute infection and nearly died;

Paul and other believers despaired for his life.[18] Timothy, who was like a son to Paul, was advised by Paul to take a little wine for a stomach disorder.[19]

Lastly, Trophimus, a Gentile Christian from Ephesus and a travelling companion of Paul's, did not accompany Paul and Luke on a particular journey because Paul informed Timothy, he left Trophimus sick at Miletus.[20]

One can't help wondering why these close associates of Paul, who healed so many others, found neither miraculous nor medical methods effective in their own circumstances.[21] Surely prayer would have been offered up to God in each of these instances for healing and recovery. But perhaps these examples are included to help us realize that we may pray to God and ask for healing and restoration; however, in God's sovereignty, as in the examples of Job and Paul, there may be reasons we don't yet understand as to why God's answer may be "no" or "not yet" regarding healing.

Ultimately, we see the apostles continuing in the ministry of Jesus as He taught and demonstrated for them and as the disciples had practiced while Jesus was still with them. Their ministry was about proclaiming the gospel of Jesus Christ coming among us to inaugurate the reign of God and gather believers into communities. Their ministry included preaching and healing as a demonstration of Jesus' loving and compassionate care. The apostles, through their faithful obedience, passed the ministry of Jesus Christ on to their followers.

Chapter 6

HEALING FROM THE EARLY CHURCH TO THE REFORMATION

We have heard it with our ears, O God; our ancestors
have told us what you did in their days, in days long
ago.

—PSALM 44:1

Christians have argued that the healing ministry of Jesus ceased after the death of the eyewitness disciples and apostles. However, there is ample evidence that, along with the proclamation of the Good News of Jesus Christ, healing continued to be part of the ministry of the Early Church.

By referring to literature written by the Early Church fathers, we know that, like Paul, they were convinced that the Good News of Christ's resurrection was at the heart of their faith and included the redemption of the whole person from every form of bondage. The flesh, as well as the spirit, was redeemed by Christ from death and every form of death, including disease. This redemption could be appropriated by every believer from the moment of their incorporation into the body of Christ, that is, their baptism.[22]

From that time on, both body and soul shared the victory of the risen Christ over sin and death. This life of victory was sustained, or restored if necessary, by the sacraments. Exorcism, holy anointing, the laying on of hands, the prayers of the church, and the invocation of Christ's name were in regular use for bringing about this restoration.[23]

Words of Our Forefathers

One of the earliest known Christian Apologies outside of the New Testament was written by Quadratus (circa 125). In it, he wrote:

> Our Saviour's works...were always present: for they were real [consisting of] those who had been healed of their diseases, those who had been raised from the dead; who were not only seen whilst they were being healed and raised up, but were [afterwards] constantly present. Nor did they remain only during the sojourn of the Saviour [on earth], but also a considerable time after his departure; and, indeed, some of them have survived even down to our own times.[24]

In *The Shepherd of Hermas* (circa 140), the author believed that the attempt to relieve the pain of the suffering was a great joy, but should not necessarily be considered praiseworthy or noteworthy; rather, he said the failure to attempt to free them was a grievous sin.[25]

Justin Martyr (circa 150–155), in speaking on the gifts of the Spirit, wrote in his *Dialogue with Trypho* that the gift of healing was still being received in his time.[26] In his *Second Apology*, he wrote of Christians who had been healed and were continuing to heal in the name of Jesus.[27]

Considered one of the most valuable sources of evidence on healing outside of the New Testament is the work of Irenaeus (circa 180). In his treatise, *Against Heresies*, Irenaeus dealt with questions regarding the claims of heretics. In response, Irenaeus wrote about the abundant evidence of healings performed by Christians. Among them were: giving sight to the blind, hearing to the deaf, casting out all sorts of demons, curing the weak, the lame, the paralytic, those distressed in any part of the body, effectually remedying external accidents, and frequently raising the dead.[28]

Irenaeus wrote that these miracles of healing were well known to his pagan readers and were performed upon Christians as well as non-Christians. The latter often became believers as a result of their healing. He attributed all these miracles to the power of God. The apostles received this power through prayer, and the church of his day, "receiving grace from Him," performed the miracles "according to the gift which each one has received from Him."[29] Such miracles were daily occurrences and were employed by the laying on of hands, invoking the name of our Lord Jesus Christ, and prayer and fasting by the entire church.[30]

In Origen's writings (martyred circa 253), there is also considerable evidence of physical healing in the Church of his time. In his work, *Against Celsus*, Origen wrote about the still-present power of Jesus, which "up to the present time still produces conversion and amelioration of life in those who believe in God through Him." He went on to write of the many cures performed by Christians through direct prayer to God, which he considered a higher way than recourse to a physician.[31]

However, the Church was about to experience an event that would massively change its course throughout history. This was the victory of Constantine the Great, who became a convert to Christianity and used his power to promote its beliefs within the Roman Empire. Most notably was the Edict of Milan in 313 A.D., which instituted a new policy of religious tolerance and began a period of governmental favour toward the church.

From a persecuted church, Christianity became not only an accepted religion, but also, and quite quickly, became the established religion of the empire. While this religious freedom was a gift in some ways, soon the church was flooded with nominal Christians who discovered that membership now brought favour and prestige. Morton Kelsey observes that this kind of climate generally does not generate enthusiasm and commitment—or works of healing. Yet within at least large parts of the church, there remained vitality of faith and dedication, and where this was so, records show that healings continued as before.[32]

A Change of Heart Toward Healing

However, as the Church's new status opened a new chapter, new priorities arose for theologians to deal with. The church had to rework not only its theology, but also "its ethics, its educational methods and its political theory in order to develop a secure intellectual base," if it were to survive its adoption by emperors.[33]

The development of Augustine's thought, through his writing, holds special interest for the understanding of Christian healing. For nearly a thousand years, Augustine was considered one of the leading theologians of the church. In his early writings, he stated quite specifically that Christians were not to look for the continuation of the gift of healing. Yet, some forty years later, toward the end of his life and shortly before he completed his last and greatest work *The City of God* in 426, Augustine had a change of heart brought about by his own experiences. In the final section of that book, he wrote about miracles of healing that occurred in his own diocese of Hippo Regius:

> I realized how many miracles were occurring in our own day and which were so like the miracles of old and also how wrong it would be to allow the memory of these marvels of divine power to perish from among our people. It is only two years ago that the keeping of records was begun here in

Hippo, and already, at this writing, we have nearly seventy attested miracles.[34]

The Difference a Wording Can Make

Another influential church father, Jerome (340–420), in writing about the subject of healing, wrote that it was not part of his own experience, yet he knew of healings from the lives of others and accepted the reality of such experiences.

His most noted contribution to Christianity was the Vulgate, a great work of scholarship, which made the Bible available in the common tongue of the Western church. It was through this work, specifically Jerome's "use of the strictly theological word salvo to translate both 'save' and 'cure'...[that] he helped to turn the church's attention away from healing, focusing it rather on what healing represented symbolically."[35]

Explaining the Decline

It's difficult to pinpoint exactly when and why the decline in healing ministries within the Church occurred, but theologian Morton Kelsey, after having struggled with this question for twenty years, has identified three trends that he believes contributed to the continuing decline of healing as part of the church's official ministry:

> First, there was a subtle and gradual alteration in the popular view of the nature of God and of humanity. This was associated with the decline of civilization in the West and the barbarian conquests.
>
> Second, there was a major shift in theological thinking...which resulted in a theology which had little place for any direct and natural contact between God and human beings, hence little room for healing.

Third, throughout these years people continued to believe in the miraculous and exhibited a lively and uncritical interest in healing miracles. Separated from theological understanding and criticism, this became more and more fanciful until it was difficult to believe many of the stories told during this period.[36]

The Church Meets the Scientific Method

Beate Jakob, the German doctor and theologian mentioned earlier, also suggests several possible reasons for the decline of healing in the ministry of the Christian Church.

One has to do with advances in medicine and the gradual claim of the medical profession over health matters. Another is that contact with popular philosophy of the day increasingly challenged Christianity to prove itself, with the result that Christian theology developed affinities toward the humanities. Christian salvation increasingly began to be seen from an intellectual point of view and was interpreted as a doctrine and a teaching.

Still another reason is that Christianity, under the influence of Greek philosophy, developed a negative attitude toward the body, with a resulting resignation toward suffering. Perhaps because of the tendency of limiting salvation to the spiritual, Christians interpreted Jesus' compassion for the sick into care for the sick, personally and communally.[37]

Henry Wildeboer, a Christian Reformed pastor, in his book on miracles, suggests some other possible reasons for the decline in the healing ministry of the Christian Church:

Though miracles were very much a part of the ancient world, the renaissance and enlightenment, along with the reformation, elevated rational thought and the scientific method. It was not respectable for scholarly people to be unable to explain unique events that were at least unnatural if not miraculous. Thus explanations abounded, arguments ensued, debates raged, and miracles seemingly decreased as discussions increased.[38]

It was, more or less, into this world that the Protestant Reformation emerged and changed many aspects of church life and practice, most notably through a return to the primacy of the Scriptures.

The Influence of an Important Few on Healing

Two of the Reformation's great theologians, Martin Luther (1483–1546) and John Calvin (1509–1564), spoke out against the possibility of healing in their day, perhaps as a way of explaining the reality of the church at that time. They saw no one raised from the dead and they saw no miraculous healing of the sick.[39]

Morton Kelsey sums up their views as "God's having given a special dispensation for these mighty works only for a particular period and purpose."[40] Martin Luther concluded that the real gift of the Holy Spirit is to enlighten Scripture, for, as Kelsey explains:

> ...now that the apostles have preached the Word and have given their writings, and nothing more than what they have written remains to be revealed, no new and special revelation or miracle is necessary.[41]

Calvin also strongly believed that the extraordinary gifts or miracles of the Holy Spirit ceased with the apostolic age. According to Calvin, God's purpose for miracles was to accredit the Word, its doctrines and its first proclaimers.[42] He argued:

But that gift of healing, like the rest of the miracles, which the Lord willed to be brought forth for a time, has vanished away in order to make the new preaching of the gospel marvellous forever. Therefore, even if we grant to the full that anointing was a sacrament of those powers which were then administered by the hands of the apostles, it now has nothing to do with us, to whom the administering of such powers has not been committed.[43]

Calvin acknowledged God's presence at all times, yet at the same time seemed to ridicule those who believed in the gift of healing:

Therefore, they make themselves ridiculous when they boast that they are endowed with the gift of healing. The Lord is indeed present with his people in every age; and he heals their weaknesses as often as necessary, no less than of old; still he does not put forth these manifest powers, nor dispense miracles through the apostles' hands. For that was a temporary gift, and also quickly perished partly on account of men's ungratefulness.[44]

As Kelsey notes, the influence of these two reformers on Protestantism can hardly be stressed enough. Benjamin B. Warfield, a professor following Calvin's thought at Princeton centuries later, was just one theologian that picked up and emphatically reinforced the cessationists' perspective.

Through his work, *Counterfeit Miracles*, published in 1918, he became one of the most prominent exponents of cessationism since Luther and Calvin themselves. However, in his work, he was so convinced of the truth of his position, that he completely overlooked many Bible passages that might speak otherwise. Among the New

Testament passages that attest to the promise of the continuation of the gifts of the Spirit, theologian Jon M. Ruthven includes I Corinthians 1:4–8 and 13:8–13; from Ephesians, 1:13–23, 3:14–21, 4:11–13, 4:30, 5:15–19, and 6:10–20; and Philippians 1:5–10.[45]

The impact of Warfield's polemic against the continuation of these gifts was massive. We might include it among the reasons that all the gifts of the Spirit gradually ceased to flow freely in the communal life of the Christian Church.

Another possible reason that some of the spiritual gifts, like healing, almost ceased to operate within the Church of Jesus Christ might have to do with the way church history is recorded.

Gary B. McGee comments on the way the history of missions is recorded and passed on in a recent article on missions. He cites two mission stories: one about Alexander Duff, a renowned Scottish missionary to India, who wrote in 1839 that "Missionaries of the Church of Scotland have been sent forth...in the absence of miracles."

The other story is about missionaries Jonathan and Deborah Wade, who worked in Burma (now Myanmar) around the same time. They lost their way in the mountains of Burma until they came upon a Karen house.

Sitting on the verandah, an elderly Karen man quietly watched them and then called out, "The teacher has arrived; the teacher has arrived!" The crowd that soon gathered had received a prophecy telling them that "the teacher is in the jungle, and will call on you. You must...listen to his precepts." The gospel was warmly received, many converts were baptized, and a permanent mission station was set up.[46]

McGee points out the fact that the former story is often recounted in mission histories, while few have heard about the miraculous events of the latter. Even though there's ample precedent for the occurrence of the miraculous in missions from the time of the apostles, there has been disagreement over their credibility. In this sense, the history of the church reflects its reality and reinforces it, erasing the memory of God's gracious and miraculous intervention, and casting doubt on its reality.

Christ came to inaugurate the reign of God among us, so that we might have life and have it abundantly, and freely seeks to bestow spiritual gifts on all believers for the mutual benefit and wellbeing of all until his return. It seems that we've not always understood or believed. In many ways, we may have inhibited the flow and the use of God's gifts. Believing in and living as heirs of the reign of God could help the church be more open to the free flowing of the Holy Spirit's gifts so that Christ's Church may once again be a true healing community for the soul as well as the body.

The Healing Continues

As we've seen, few practices within Christianity have had a more legitimate ancestry than praying for the healing of the sick in the context of the proclamation of the Good News of Jesus Christ.

The tradition of divine healing within the Church has been long and well-documented. Christians in all ages of the Church's history have prayed for and believed in the miraculous intervention of God to heal. At times, the practice has been normative in the life of the church, as in the Apostolic Church and the Early Church, but at other periods, healing ministries existed mainly on the periphery of the church.[47]

Chapter 7

THE RE-EMERGENCE
OF A MOVEMENT

My son, if you accept my words and store up my com-
mands within you, turning your ear to wisdom and
applying your heart to understanding—indeed, if you
call out for insight and cry aloud for understanding,
and if you look for it as for silver and search for it as
for hidden treasure, then you will understand the fear
of the Lord and find the knowledge of God. For the
Lord gives wisdom; from his mouth come knowledge
and understanding.
—PROVERBS 2:1–6

Among the historical forefathers of more recent and modern charismatic movements were several religious movements that included the belief and practice of healing as part of their ministry.

Among them were the Society of Friends, or Quakers, who had
migrated to America from England in the mid-seventeenth century.
Their founder, George Fox, had a significant healing ministry and
travelled around America in 1672. Many healings in response to
prayer and laying on of hands were reported and recorded. Fox always insisted that their healing was under the divine sovereignty of

God and if healings didn't happen immediately following the prayer of faith, the person was not chastised for lack of faith.

The Quakers also demonstrated their confidence in both medicine and medical doctors. Instances of divine healings were not regarded as proofs of their ministry. Rather, they were seen as being a part of their total ministry.[48]

For John Wesley, leader of the Methodists, healings were not a central theme in his ministry, yet he recorded several events that we might call "miraculous." Among Pietists, Dayton notes, "their biblical realism and pastoral orientation combined with a belief in the continuation of miracles and produced a doctrine of healing through prayer and faith."[49]

One figure who is significant for this study and is of the Reformed tradition is minister Andrew Murray from South Africa. In the late eighteenth century, he was "among the most prominent and significant individuals to receive physical healing at Bethshan," a faith home in London, established to accommodate those seeking healing.[50]

Murray wrote that "after being stopped for more than two years of my ministry, I was healed by the mercy of God in answer to the prayer of those who see in *Him 'the Lord that healeth thee'*" (Exodus 15:26).

He went on to express what a source of rich spiritual blessing his healing was to him and how he clearly came to see "that the Church possesses in Jesus, our Divine Healer, an inestimable treasure, which she does not yet know how to appreciate."[51]

In response to his experience and subsequent study of the Scriptures, Murray felt he could no longer keep silent, and published a series of meditations to show, according to the Word of God, that *"the prayer of faith"* (James 5:15) is the means appointed by God for the cure of the sick. In true Reformed fashion, Murray expressed his purpose:

...to show that this truth is in perfect accord with Holy Scripture, and that the study of this truth is essential for everyone who desires to see the Lord manifest His power and His glory in the midst of His children.[52]

In a meditation on "Health and Salvation by the Name of Jesus," Murray emphasized the theme of God's power and glory:

"Wherever the Spirit acts with power, He works divine healings... If divine healing is seen but rarely in our day, we can attribute it to no other cause than that the Spirit does not act with power... It is the will of God to glorify His Son in the Church, and He will do it wherever He finds faith."[53]

Healing and the Anglican Church

The Anglicans have had a "Rite of Healing" in *The Book of Common Prayer* since the sixteenth century.[54] Donald W. Dayton, in tracing Pentecostal roots in the Methodist tradition, makes an interesting comment about John Wesley's Anglican roots, for "through his parents Wesley was a product of the high church Anglican tradition with its tendency to preserve a doctrine of the miraculous."[55]

Today, many churches in the Anglican tradition offer anointing and prayer for healing following the Eucharist as well as during special healing services. Several books have been published in recent years by those involved, witnessing to the healing work of God in response to prayer and special healing ministries. The International Order of St. Luke the Physician comes out of that tradition and has had an impact on many.

In 1960, Francis MacNutt was teaching at a seminary in Iowa when he was invited to a nearby Presbyterian seminary to attend a lecture. There he heard Alfred Price speak on healing. The passage Price spoke from was from Matthew 10:1 and 5–8a, taken from the New Revised Standard Version (NRSV):

"Then Jesus summoned his twelve disciples and gave them authority over unclean spirits, to cast them out, and to cure every disease and every sickness... These twelve Jesus sent out with the following instructions: 'Go nowhere among the Gentiles, and enter no town of the Samaritans, but go rather to the lost sheep of the house of Israel. As you go, proclaim the good news, "The kingdom of heaven has come near." Cure the sick, raise the dead, cleanse the lepers, cast out demons.'"

At that time, MacNutt was a member of an order that based its ministry on this very passage. They had been taught to do the first part—to go and proclaim the Good News—but the other part they had never been taught to do.

They were asked that day why they thought they could preach and not also think they could heal the sick and cast out evil spirits. And that, suggests MacNutt, is the basic question to ask the Church. He credits the ministry of the Order of St. Luke with the fact that it's no longer strange for healing to occur in the church, not only in North America but around the world, something that was not at all true in 1960.[56]

MacNutt and many others continue to write, teach, and lead healing services in many churches. He believes that Christian believers in general have been deprived of the riches of the gospel. Even though only some have the gift of healing, all Christians can be used by God. All Christians need to be encouraged to pray with and for their families, as well as in the church, for healing and wholeness.

An Ongoing Discomfort

Wildeboer, in his book on healing, suggests some reasons for the continued reluctance of many mainline churches to once again embrace a public healing ministry:

In orderly evangelical and Reformed churches, healing ministries—especially exorcisms—are often associated with fringe areas of the Christian church. It is not part of our more sophisticated congregational life. For many generations, healings and exorcisms were associated with inner-city, store-front Pentecostal churches where maximum ardor and minimum order prevailed. Where orderliness takes top priority, where spontaneity is feared, and where disorderliness is a threat, miracles and healings rarely occur.[57]

Healing Here and Now

Regarding the gift of healing, Paul lists it as a specific gift given only to some. James, on the other hand, assigns to the church elders the task of praying for the sick, anointing them with oil in the name of the Lord, because "the prayer of faith will save the sick, and the Lord will raise them up."[58]

One of the regular tasks of pastors is to visit the sick and pray with and for them. Every church can testify to answers to such prayers, whether healing comes through the skills of a physician or medication, or whether such healing can't be explained by the medical profession. In every case, thanksgiving and praise belong to God.[59]

Spiritual or divine healing, once central to the ministry of the Christian Church, is not only a real possibility, but is once again becoming a very present reality in many parts of the Body of Jesus Christ.

Chapter 8

MENTAL HEALTH HEARTACHE

I waited patiently for the Lord; he turned to me and
heard my cry. He lifted me out of the slimy pit, out of
the mud and mire; he set my feet on a rock and gave
me a firm place to stand. He put a new song in my
mouth, a hymn of praise to our God. Many will see and
fear the Lord and put their trust in him.
—PSALM 40:1–3

Merlyn Persaud was just sixteen years old when she met the man who would become her husband, and only eighteen years old when she married him. Young and full of optimism for the future, they soon had a beautiful baby girl, settled into an idyllic home of their own, and secured jobs they felt confident in. Everything was going according to plan.

Merlyn got pregnant again, and things seemed to be going just as smoothly as they had with their daughter. However, when the child was born, doctors told Merlyn that the child was intellectually disabled, and that his life would be a string of one medical issue after another. Merlyn was devastated. She thought their lives were over.

The family moved in with Merlyn's Christian in-laws for the first couple weeks. Merlyn was struggling intensely and suffered a nervous breakdown soon after the birth. "I would cry myself to sleep, then I would wake up gripped with fear of the future," she remembers. "What were we going to do? What was going to happen? How am I, at the age of twenty-two, and my husband at twenty-four, how were we going raise [this] child?"

But the family helped keep them going. Merlyn's mother-in-law would sleep in the same room and woke up early every morning to lay her hand on the baby's forehead and pray for him. In the evenings, when her father-in-law returned home from work, the entire family would gather around the baby and sing the old hymn, "The Great Physician." But eventually Merlyn and her husband and children re-settled in their own home and began trying to navigate their new life.

Raising their son, Daniel Paul, was not an easy task. To add to his health and cognitive struggles, Daniel Paul also exhibited difficult and aggressive behaviours, making it impossible for the family to find care for him. One parent had to stay home at all times whenever the other went out. However, when Merlyn's husband came to a saving faith a while into their marriage, he decided he wanted to go along with the rest of his family to church Sunday mornings. The only option was to bring Daniel Paul along.

Can Church Attendance Affect Healing?

"I didn't know how that was going to work because of his behaviour problems," Merlyn admits. "We took him to church the first, the second week and instantaneously the [aggressive] behaviour stopped. He calmed right down." Almost interrupting herself, she says with warmth, "And he's a loving boy. He loves people. He loves music. He loves going for drives. He has a good appetite. He loves going for burgers. And he's a really, wonderful, lovely child."

Though today he struggles with frequent ankle injuries, his health, overall wellness, and general disposition otherwise are quite good, something for which Merlyn credits God.

"It's easy to say, 'What have I done, that you've given me this child? Is it something that I've done wrong that you're punishing me?' But I heard someone say to see it from the opposite side," Merlyn says, welling up with emotion. "Maybe God chooses special parents. He sees something in my husband and I that made Him choose us to raise Daniel Paul. Then having a child [with special needs] is not a punishment; it's actually a privilege."

Merlyn is full of gratefulness over all she and her family have learned from their son. Through raising him, they've learned sacrifice and selflessness, humility, and perseverance, and how to come together as a family in whatever trials face them. Perhaps highest of all, they've learned unconditional love. They've grown a passion for loving those society so easily ignores, for whatever reason that may be, and this heart for unconditionally loving all people drives them on in their ministry.

So, after many years of struggle, the family seemed settled into life with their son and were even doing so with joy and thankfulness. But when things finally seemed stable with Daniel Paul, Merlyn began facing an even more personal challenge.

"I was on the mountain top. I was working for National Defense and had just received a promotion. We had started a home church that I was pastoring. And I decided I wanted to go to school to get ordained," Merlyn continues. "Daniel Paul was doing well. My daughters were doing well, and they were right there along with us in the ministry. We were excited. I had everything all planned. School, then retirement from my job and ministry full-time, even our mortgage would be paid off. They were grooming me at work to do counselling, so even though it was unheard of, my workplace offered to pay for some of the courses at the Christian college I was going to. Everything was in my favour."

The Frightening Fall into Mental Illness

But suddenly things took a turn. "I don't know what happened. I just started to feel tired and have problems coping. I couldn't keep up with my workload. I couldn't keep up with the house. And I couldn't understand why.

"Suddenly I felt like people were following me. Cars are following me. They've bugged the house. People are coming to kill me, to kill my daughters, and to kill my husband." She continues. "I was sitting at home with my husband and daughter, and I told them, 'Do you hear that? They bugged the house. They bugged the house.' And they didn't know what was happening. They thought I had schizophrenia.

"When we got to the doctor's office, I thought they were going to put me in an institution. This was all part of the psychosis. I ran out of the doctor's office and I started running out on the road to get away. [My family] ran out of the doctor's office and ran behind me. I was steps away from the highway, and my husband ran behind me, and he held on to me as they called the police. I reached down and bit him. I thought my life was over. What I was going through, it's hard to explain.

"The police came and took me to the hospital where I was diagnosed with psychosis. Immediately, they put me on medication. And I started to recover. I went back to work. I took a break from school. And everything was okay. I felt great. I bounced right back."

After three months, Merlyn decided she felt good enough to go back to school, only to experience a psychotic episode there a short time later. Changes to her medication and an easing of responsibilities saw her beginning to recover again. After nine months, she decided to try school again, only to have another psychotic episode and land back at square one once again. This particularly severe episode kept her in the hospital for five weeks.

Merlyn reflects on her experience and explains, "Whatever's happening to you, it feels just as real as me talking to you. With this more severe attack, the doctors decided it was not only psychotic, it was severe depression with psychotic features. So I ended up back on several medications and they deemed that I couldn't go back to work. The doctors said, 'No ministry, no school, no work.'

"Psychosis affects your concentration, your comprehension, your memory, and the depression kills your desire. The desire to read, the desire to pray, the desire to go out, to socialize, to interact, even to maintain your personal hygiene. It killed all those desires. You just want to lay there." She goes on, "In an instant, I had lost everything. My ability to drive was affected by the psychosis, so I lost my job, where I had just got a promotion. I lost my ministry, and school, which I loved. I lost all my dreams, all my plans, everything was shattered.

"But the thing I lost the most with psychosis was my desire to pray, to read—that love and that intimacy, that passion and that zeal and that fire that I had for the Lord and for ministry. All of it was gone. I would go to church, and before I would lift my hand and pray and worship and cry, I had such a bond and a closeness and an intimacy. Now I would go to church and just stand, there completely numb.

"But I have to say that, it's been six years, and gradually it's coming back. I've been fighting it. Even if I can't pray a long prayer, I'll force myself to say a short prayer that may just consist of, 'Lord help me.' Or, 'Lord hold my hand again. Lord, give me faith, give me courage, give me strength.' When I read the Bible, I don't read a whole chapter. I may read just a little bit of the Psalms, which is a good place to start when you're struggling through a hard time. I take it a verse at a time. I meditate on that one verse, and it ministers to my soul. I also have worship music going on in the house. Right now, I'm completely dependent on Him. I'm completely relying on Him. He has to carry me, because I need Him now."

Merlyn admits, "I had my days when I said, 'God, You betrayed me. You left me. You abandoned me. You don't love me. You don't care about me. All my dreams, You took everything from me. But the mere fact that I'm doing this interview shows that God had a greater plan from what even I saw. If my testimony can impact just one person, if it could give somebody hope and strength and encouragement; if it's just one person I can speak to, it would be worth it.

She stops and adds, "It's not easy pastoring our small church, or raising a child [with special needs], and fighting depression and psychosis. And we had the usual problems a marriage would have: marital problems, financial problems, etc. My testimony is by no means that we've come out of all of it. We're going through it. We're going through it right now. And we're taking it not a day at a time, we're taking it by the moment. Anything can change in a day. We're taking it moment by moment. And we're relying on the Lord to help us."

"If You're Going Through Hell, Keep Going"

When we seem to have reached the depths of despair, it can be easy to want to stop moving forward, to instead just sit down and wallow in our self-pity. Maybe we even want to give up on life in a more dramatic, irreversible way. Winston Churchill's above quote seems to imply there's another side, an eventual escape from the desperate situation we're going through. But what if we're not sure there is? What if the road ahead is long, and we're not sure things will ever change?

There's a story of a man who came home from church one day, discouraged. As he had been sitting listening to the sermon, he realized, "For over fifty years, I've been coming to church every single Sunday, and I cannot say I clearly remember a single sermon. Maybe bits and pieces and themes, but that's it. Has all this just been a waste of time then?"

The man wrestled with the question all afternoon until he sat down to supper. As he was sitting with his wife, enjoying her food, he had a realization. He realized that, for decades, his wife had been preparing him meals. While he enjoyed her cooking and could rattle of the kinds of dishes she made, he could not necessarily recall specific meals. He wasn't able to tell you what she made if you requested the information for a certain date, nor could he comment on subtle changes from one roast beef to the next. And yet, if he had started ignoring the meals altogether and skipping out on them because he couldn't remember them, he would have died.

Even though no meal had been particularly impactful in a life-altering way, their continued presence had sustained him and given him life all those years. And so it was with the practice of listening to sermons. Though he could not link specific lessons with specific Sundays, the truths he heard each week had sustained him in his faith all those years, keeping him spiritually alive and growing deeper in his faith.

This lesson applies to all spiritual disciplines and is perhaps especially true during times of despair. Like Merlyn, at such times, it is often the case that we feel dry and numb spiritually, and it can be hard to be motivated to carry on our usual spiritual practices. We may feel like they're making no impact and that there's therefore no point in forcing ourselves to do something that just feels like pulling teeth. But that's not even remotely true.

"What has kept me has been the Word of God," says Merlyn. "I read 2 Timothy, which says, 'When you're faithless, He is faithful.' So, even if I have just a little bit of faith to hold on and not to give up, that's enough. The Word of God has been the source of my strength."

She continues, "If I had to say one thing to somebody [who's] going through the deep dark black hole that is depression right now, or who's going through psychosis, or any mental illness, I would say, 'Hold on.' The Bible says, '...*for though the righteous fall seven times...*' (Proverbs 24:16, NIV). You're gonna fall, it's going to happen. But you know what, you get back up.

"And pray. Even if you don't feel like it, pray. Even if you can just pray, 'God help me.' He's close to the brokenhearted, and He will never leave you or forsake you. Just hold on to the words that, whatever He started in you, He'll finish."

With all that, Merlyn and her family have gone through, there must have been many times that it seemed doubtful that they could move back into a life of joy, peace, and normal family togetherness. But Merlyn holds on to hope, and the evidence that it's well-founded:

"One by one, I've started to come off the medication. I'm off the depression medication. I'm off the anxiety medication. I'm still on the psychosis medication, but one by one, I'm coming off of them."

Merlyn had one set of ideas about what her life would look like, but, "God had a bigger plan. Though at the time, we didn't see it. My husband and I started a church and a ministry, and people ask us, 'Why are you doing what you're doing? Why would you take on such a big responsibility?'

"And we say to them, 'Our son has taught us to love others. He gave us a compassion for souls that makes us want to reach out to people. We want to help people. We want to tell people about God who has been the source of our strength and our health. And raising him has taught us to rely on God. Without Him, we can't do it. We can't do it alone, we can't do it without His help. God has been the source of our strength.'"

Chapter 9

THE LONGING FOR
A CHILD

But those who hope in the Lord will renew their
strength. They will soar on wings like eagles; they will
run and not grow weary, they will walk and not be faint.
—ISAIAH 40:31

When Bill and Aymie were married in May of 2013, Aymie was
ready to have children right away. After a year of trying, the
couple started to wonder if something was wrong, and Aymie's doctor
referred her to a specialist. After a review of her health, the doctor
began to suspect Aymie had endometriosis, a condition that has treatments, but no definite cure.

Aymie remembers, "It was hard to walk through that, particularly because it's not just one disappointment for you to get over, but
it happens month after month after month. At the beginning of the
month, you start with so much hope that this could be it, maybe this
month it could happen. And as you wait, it's hard not to read into
every symptom that you have, thinking, 'Is this different, could this
possibly be it?' It's almost embarrassing to say the amount of pregnancy tests I took. If I could have willed the baby into existence, it would

have been there. But it wasn't. It was an emotional rollercoaster, and it was very emotionally draining."

She continues, "I think it's really easy to think, 'God, where are you? Why me?' But it's not necessarily about what you did right or wrong; we live in a fallen world, so things happen. God didn't promise that [bad] things wouldn't happen to us; He promised He would be there with us through it all. So, we thought, 'Well God, You're the only One who can fix this, the only One who can make it better. And if we don't have You in this, we have nothing. You are bigger than the diagnosis, so we're just going to keep on going with what we're doing and believe You for a family.'"

Aymie had surgery to definitively determine whether she had endometriosis. The news wasn't good. Not only was the endometriosis extremely severe, but doctors also found a polyp inside her uterus, which meant it was a hostile environment for an embryo to implant. The couple were devastated and so in disbelief that they asked for a retest. But even after praying and fasting and believing that the polyp would be gone, the results were the same.

"At that point in the journey, three years in, all we had left to say to God was, 'Even if we haven't seen You as a God who heals in this situation, we know You're the God who heals. Even though we haven't seen a miracle in this situation, we know You're the God of miracles. Even though we haven't seen the impossible happen yet, we know You're the God who makes the impossible possible,'" Aymie says. "And so, even though we were so low and so exhausted, we continued to walk in surrender."

A surgery was scheduled to sort out Aymie's endometriosis and the polyp in her uterus. "I went in for my pre-op bloodwork and they said to me, 'Is there any chance you could be pregnant?' I said, 'Nope.'" Aymie goes on, "I got a call later that day from the fertility clinic. The doctor said, 'We have to cancel your surgery. Aymie, you're pregnant.'"

Aymie describes what it was like to receive the news. "We were completely shocked. I was actually driving with my friend and my doctor was on speaker phone. When she told me, I said, 'Oh my gosh! I have to pull over, wait just a second!' My friend was beside me in the car trying not to scream. It was probably one of the best moments of my life."

From One Blessing to Another

Aymie describes the daughter who came into their lives nine months later: "Lyra is the best thing. She is smart, active, sensitive, and she loves to read. She loves to learn, she loves to run, she loves for us to play. She's a total mama's girl. Lyra, her name, means 'song of pure joy' and I feel that it really describes her character."

But Lyra wasn't the last blessing God had in store for Bill and Aymie. "When Lyra was almost a year old, we thought maybe we could start trying for a second [child]," Aymie explains. "We had braced ourselves for a long journey, for the long haul. It had been three years the first time, and we didn't know how long the second could possibly take or if this was going to be another journey of infertility and trusting God and believing for a second child. But just five months later, we became pregnant. We are currently expecting our second child in January, and we just found out it's a boy."

Since their wrestling with infertility, faith, and discouragement, Bill and Aymie have been basking in the joy of parenthood. But they haven't forgotten the valley that God brought them through.

Aymie recounts, "When we first went in for the appointment at the fertility clinic, we were told it was basically next to impossible for us to become pregnant on our own, given the diagnosis that I had and the polyp working against us. But God made the impossible possible for us. The doctor said 'no,' but God said 'yes.'"

She goes on, "I remember so much of what it's like to be at that point of absolute devastation. At my lowest point, I decided I was an atheist for all of two hours. But in the darkest moments, we chose to run to God rather than away from God because His Word says that He has good plans for us, to give us hope and a future. So we just trusted that His plans for us were good. And even if we didn't understand, even if we hadn't seen what we wanted to see, that didn't change who He was. We just completely surrendered and trusted, and that was how we coped."

Aymie pauses. "But, you know, to those who are struggling, I hope our message will encourage them to believe that God can do the impossible for them too." She nods, "What God does for one, He can do for another."

Many of us will have experienced the desire to be in someone's else shoes. Perhaps the first time was way back in your early years of school, when you envied a bike or dress or some other treasure that belonged to a classmate. Perhaps sometimes our envy also involved being rid of a burden or insufficiency we didn't feel we deserved to be burdened with. In Aymie's case, it involved her infertility and then the blessing of pregnancy.

"I remember at one point, I could count approximately twenty people [whom] I knew who had just given birth or were pregnant," she says. "It was really tough, and initially I struggled with feelings of jealousy. You want to be happy for other people, but you have so much pain from the disappointment of not being pregnant and waiting for so long."

Anyone who has had or worked with children knows "It's not fair!" is one of the first and most universal phrases to come out of our young mouths. But if wisdom doesn't intervene, this phrase can follow us all the way up into the twilight of our years.

Battling Self-Pity

When we're experiencing trials with our health, inappropriate self-pity is a very real danger. It can be a particularly tricky obstacle around which to navigate, because there's a need for us to be honest with what we're feeling. When we're suffering intense health problems, it's to be expected that there will be feelings of fear, pain, loss, confusion, and exhaustion. The situation you may be going through is, in all likelihood, legitimately extremely difficult, and having heavy feelings related to it is completely valid. However, it's possible to have these feelings arise and to deal with them without resorting to self-pity.

Elisabeth Elliot was a missionary for several years in Ecuador. She and her husband, Jim, had waited long to marry, feeling at first that it wasn't God's will or timing for them. Finally, after five years, they felt that God gave them the green light. The two were married just over two years and had just had a baby girl when Jim was murdered by the very people to whom they had gone to preach the gospel.

Though Elisabeth was sure she would never be able to marry again, after many years, she did fall in love and became a wife for a second time. But not long after the wedding, her husband was diagnosed with a very fast-acting cancer and died a very painful, difficult death.

If anyone had a right to self-pity, it was Elisabeth. And yet, you will scarcely find anyone more intentionally guarded against self-pity than her. "I know of nothing more paralyzing, more deadly, than self-pity," she once wrote.[60]

She knew that self-pity can be a terribly enticing temptation and trap to fall into; at first, it seems to be a balm to our wounds, a sweetly validating acknowledgment of our pain that comforts us by appealing to our wounded pride and intrinsic tendency toward self-centredness.

But though self-pity may at first seem like the warm arms of a mother stroking her child's face with a tender "There, there," in a moment it flips the switch and swiftly tightens those arms around our throats to suffocate us. And it does so by taking our eyes off Christ and placing them on ourselves, then on the comparison of ourselves with those around us.

"Comparison is the thief of joy," Eleanor Roosevelt famously once said, and this is exactly what we find in cases of self-pity. What seems like a delicious momentary indulgence and temporary relief will end up clawing us by the throat and pulling us down out of the reach of all hope, joy, peace, perspective, and truth.

According to Elisabeth Elliot, who quite likely knew the temptation intimately herself, "[Self-pity] is a death that has no resurrection, a sinkhole from which no rescuing hand can drag you, because you have chosen to sink."[61]

But the problem remains that our pain is there, often both physically and emotionally. How are we to deal with longings unfulfilled, futures uncertain, and dreams taken away?

We must always start with turning our eyes on Jesus. Though this may seem like a vague and meaningless platitude, it is, in all truth, the best and only starting place. The Psalms are a perfect example of this. David and the other Psalmists were constantly in circumstances that had them writhing with despair, discouragement, and desperation. But perhaps it was in the very process of bringing these emotions to throne of his Saviour that David became a man after God's own heart (1 Samuel 13:14).

Like him, we must come to God's throne and pour out our hearts to Him, both the beautiful and the ugly, the confidence and the confusion. As Jacob did, we must not be afraid to wrestle with God, refusing to let Him go until we have received our blessing. Practically, this may mean getting down on your knees and weeping out your exasperation in prayer, having a prayer journal, or even having a friend come beside you who will point you to truth as you confess the frustration and lies you are tempted to believe. Likely a mix of all three strategies will be helpful.

And though it can feel like "tough love" at first, by forcefully fixing our eyes on the sufferings of Christ and tearing them away from our own sufferings, we are brought into a place of perspective, acceptance, and kinship with Christ. Elisabeth Elliot writes:

> It is one thing to call a spade a spade, to acknowledge that this thing is indeed suffering. It's no use telling yourself it's nothing. When Paul called it a 'slight' affliction, he meant it only by comparison with the glory. But it's another thing to regard one's own suffering as uncommon, or disproportionate, or undeserved. What have 'deserts' got to do with anything? We are all under the Mercy, and Christ knows the precise weight and proportion of our sufferings—He bore them. He carried our sorrows. He suffered, wrote George Macdonald, not that we might not suffer, but that our sufferings might be like His. To hell, then, with self-pity.[62]

"Do the Next Thing"

So how do we deal with the day-to-day waiting, once we've poured out our hearts to God and have resolved to fight off self-pity? The ever-practical Elisabeth Elliot has a beautifully simple answer for us here.

In a line taken from an old Saxon poem, she would simply advise people to "Do the next thing."[63] When we're in a place of suffering, we can be tempted to lethargically wallow our days away, both due to the weight of our pain, and because what once just seemed to be the normal tasks of the day now seem to be an overwhelming mountain of obstacles we could never imagine we'd have the strength to climb.

But if we're just lying around, wallowing, marinating in our darkness until we're fully saturated with it, we are not helping our physical, emotional, or spiritual health. Sometimes the everyday tasks God has ordained for us to do can be a great blessing, giving our mind a break by occupying it with practical duties instead of forcing it to keep fighting the self-pity and bitterness that keep knocking on its door. And by just focusing on one task at a time, and taking satisfaction in completing that one task, we will not be overwhelmed into lethargy by our entire "to-do" list.

For example, you may very well know all the items you have on the list, but for now, just focus on the next thing—the dishes. Once you're finished, take a moment of satisfaction in that. Then move on; what is the next task to be accomplished? It could very well be that your illness won't allow you to do as much as you once could, but that isn't something to concern yourself with while you are doing what you *can* do.

At the end of the day, don't think of your to-do list as having a bunch of unchecked boxes; instead, think of having started the day off with a blank page on which you've written down all you *were* able to do today, things that would have otherwise gone undone. Focus not on what you weren't able to do, but on all that you were. Those are things you've already taken off the list for tomorrow, so when you wake up, you've already got a head start!

Aymie was able to go one step further and set herself to a task that directly attacked her self-pity. She tells the story: "To deal with the disappointment, I began crocheting baby blankets for other pregnant women. I decided that, until I was pregnant myself and even beyond that, I would choose to bless pregnant women and that I was just going to come at it with an opposite spirit of love. I just wanted to bless other women who were pregnant and who were where I wanted to be."

Elisabeth Elliot writes:

There is nothing like definite, overt action to overcome the inertia of grief. The appearance of Joseph of Arimathea to take away the body of Jesus must have greatly heartened the other disciples, so prostrate with their own grief that they had probably not thought of doing anything at all. Nicodemus, too, thought of something he could do—he brought a mixture of myrrh and aloes—and the women who had come with Jesus from Galilee went off to prepare spices and ointments. This clear-cut action lifted them out of themselves. That is what we need in a time of crisis.

Instead of praying only for the strength we ourselves need to survive, this day or this hour, how about praying for some to give away? How about trusting God to fulfill His own promise, 'My power is made perfect in weakness'? (2 Corinthians 12:9). Where else is His power more perfectly manifested than in a human being who, well knowing his own weakness, lays hold by faith on the Strong Son of God, Immortal Love?[64]

So today, whatever we are faced with, whatever longing we wait for or weight we are praying for God to take off our back, let us look upon the cross of our Saviour, remembering that, in all things, however mysterious they may seem, God is loving us through them. Let us remember the suffering of Christ who bore the very pain we're now experiencing on the cross, and knowing all this, let us trust Him to give us the strength to "do the next thing." And when that's finished, the thing after that.

Chapter 10

ENDOMETRIOSIS, KIDNEY CORRECTION, AND RENEWAL

You intended to harm me, but God intended it for good to accomplish what is now being done, the saving of many lives.

—GENESIS 50:20

At twenty-eight years old, Carrie Hung married Tommy Tsui, a young man she had studied with in university. Shortly after their marriage, the two came to Canada to increase their scientific skills and experience with hopes of returning to Hong Kong as tentmaker missionaries. They also began hoping for a child.

But around this time, Carrie began experiencing intense and almost unbearable pains that medical tests soon attributed to two separate issues: Carrie had a lesion on her left ovary, and a polyp in her uterus. Carrie's doctors told her she could not conceive until both matters were attended to.

"It was a little disappointing and scary, too," she remembers. "I had a few friends who were doctors that told me it was very likely the polyp would be benign, but there was a chance that it could be cancerous.

"I began to get very upset and I was even angry for a while. I remember there was one day I just couldn't concentrate on my work. I was so upset that I told my boss I had to go home. I kneeled down by my bed and I started questioning God. In my anger, I confronted Him, asking, 'Why is this happening to me? God, haven't You known I've always wanted to have children of my own? I'm almost thirty; I'm not that young anymore. What kind of news is this after I just got married?'

"I was kneeling next to my bed. I had my eyes closed. And as I was pouring out all my anger to God, suddenly there was an overwhelming—I don't know how to describe it—but I quieted down at that point. Though my eyes were closed, I saw images in my mind. They were images from before I came to Canada, of the three years while I was studying for my PhD in Hong Kong with Tommy. They were images of my church, my workplace, my lab, my home, my family. Images of me behaving horribly to them. It was terrible! I hadn't realized it at the time, but I saw how badly I had behaved.

"I was very proud at church. I was very arrogant spiritually, thinking that I knew a lot more about the Bible than others, or I could sing and didn't have to practice as much as the rest. All the terrible, terrible things I had done," she continues. "I was shocked, and I was ashamed because I hadn't realized that I was such a horrible person until that point. I broke down and I stopped questioning God. I couldn't confront or condemn Him anymore because I saw myself, the ugly side of myself that I didn't know until that point. I started crying, and I remember just begging God to forgive me and to help me. I never knew I was such a horrible person, and I didn't want to be such a person. So, I cried and cried and cried. I didn't question God anymore, or even ask for healing. I just thanked God for forgiving me.

"I felt so terrible that I felt like I needed to write to my friends, my brothers and sisters, and my family," Carrie goes on. "So I took a few days of time to write to each person [who] was close to me and those [whom] I remembered I had offended in one way or another. I wrote each of them an email to apologize and ask their forgiveness. And I'm very thankful that all of them replied to me with so much grace and support. Some said they didn't even remember the offense I was apologizing for! But it was still important."

Carrie's awakening fundamentally changed her as a person. But she still had her appointment with the gynecologist ahead.

From Spiritual to Physical Healing

Carrie remembers the day clearly. "My doctor had asked me to take the month off, so at the time, I was already on my leave. I went into the building and waited patiently for my turn. When I walked into the office, the gynecologist asked me, 'So why are you here?' I replied, 'I'm here to schedule surgery with you.'"

"The doctor seemed confused. 'But what's wrong with you?'"

"So I told her my history. I gave her copies of my reports. She told me, 'But the last scan you had showed nothing. It was clear.' I was shocked and confused. 'Are you sure?' I asked her. 'Because I had three or four reports showing the same issues.' And then she asked me to wait for a minute and she called the technician [who] did the scan for me. After she hung up the phone, she just told me, 'You're good to go. There's no need for surgery.'

"I still wasn't sure what was happening," Carrie continues. "So, I just walked out of the clinic and walked to the bus stop. On my way, I was trying to figure out what was going on. I saw my family doctor regularly, and I had not one, but multiple scans, multiple images, and ultrasounds. I walked into a café and sat down there, and suddenly I realized that God had healed me.

"I was speechless. How was it possible? But if the doctor was so certain that there was nothing wrong with me, then it must have been true. I went home and told my husband that there was no need for surgery because the doctor couldn't find anything wrong; God just healed me. And he told me, 'Wait a minute. Let's not get too excited too soon. Let's wait a few months. You've had this problem for a couple of years already. Let's wait and see if this new assessment is true.'"

Tommy remembers his thinking at the time. "I had always believed that God could accomplish supernatural acts. I had read all the healing stories in the Bible, and I had no reason to doubt that Jesus had done them. I was a scientist working as a researcher, but I never really found a contradiction between the two.

"Science, by definition, is about trying to understand how natural laws are functioning, how they govern the phenomena that we observe in the natural world," he describes. "But God is outside science. God is above science. He created science, created the world, created the natural law. So I think it would be very easy for Him to twist something against the natural law once in a while, as He deems fit. But to expect it to happen to *us*, that's another story."

"[And] the pain never came back," Carrie smiles. "Since that time, I've been all good."

Carrie seemed to have experienced a miraculous healing. But her hope for children was delayed once again when another unforeseen obstacle appeared.

"Not long after this miracle, I started having fevers," Carrie explains, "Low-grade fevers [that] lasted for three weeks to a month. I think there were ten episodes of these low-grade fevers."

When Health Declines Rather Than Improves

When doctors investigated, they found the issue was related to Carrie's kidneys, bladder, and urinary tract. She was told it was a very common problem, and that there was a simple forty-five-minute surgery that could fix it. But when Carrie went in for the surgery, the procedure that was supposed to last less than an hour was extended to five. There had been complications, and after ten days in the hospital, Carrie's doctors told her that the surgery hadn't been successful.

A few temporary solutions were put in place, but eventually, another surgery would be needed. Carrie's kidney was struggling and was at risk of failing if the issue wasn't addressed soon. After a discussion of her options, the surgery date was scheduled.

"I had the imaging done two weeks before the surgery, and the doctor told me, 'You can't wait any longer, this is it.' I was actually very nervous because when the surgeon saw me outside the operating room, he told me, 'One person has died in my hands, and about seven of them have had kidney failure, but I've done this procedure a thousand times. You should be safe,'" Carrie recalls, laughing.

"He asked me to sign a consent form, and then I was left outside the operation room to be pushed into the room for surgery. I remember I was very scared," Carrie admits, but continues, "As I was waiting and wondering, I lifted my eyes and saw a cross on the door of the operation room. It was at [a Catholic hospital], so every room had a cross on the door of the room. [Suddenly], I heard a voice inside me, asking me, 'Haven't you devoted yourself to God?' And it was like someone just knocked me down and picked me up again. I said, 'Yes, that's right! Both myself and Tommy, we have dedicated our lives to God. And that also means that my body belongs to God.'

"So, at that point, I said a prayer. I said, 'God, my life and Tommy's life are Yours. And so is my body. Take it. Use it as You will.' And after saying that prayer, I felt an immense peace within me. I was no longer afraid. I just felt, 'God, I'm ready. Do whatever You have to do! My body and my life are in Your hands.' And then I was pushed into the operating room."

After going through such a struggle, Carrie was finally at peace and ready for whatever was ahead.

A Surgery Over Before It Began

"It was very strange, because I was wide awake during the whole procedure. The doctor came in and drew crosses on my tummy, where to draw a hole, I guess," Carries says, laughing again. "And then I saw a huge monitor on the wall. I could see my own organs. I remember him asking the nurse to put in a bit more dye, because he wanted to see the images more clearly. So, the nurse did.

"After a while, he came to me and asked, 'Can you tell me about your problem? Your medical history?' So I told him everything I knew about myself. And then I saw that he seemed very puzzled and deep in thought. So, I asked him, 'Didn't you see my report? I've had a lot of tests these past two weeks. My doctor told me I must have the surgery now, I can't wait.'

"He said, 'But I can't open you up. I don't see any problem with you. Your records show you had a surgery already half a year ago, but I can't even see the scar or locate any problem. And your kidney is fine.' Then he said, 'Give me one more moment, I need to talk to your urologist.'

"So, he called my urologist and talked on the phone for a few minutes. Then he came back and said, 'I'm sorry, I really can't open you up. Go home, and if there's any concern, we'll call you and ask you to come back.' The nurse was embarrassed, and she told me, 'You know we don't normally push people into the operating room and then ask them to go home.'"

Carrie's urologist followed her case with monthly appointments for three years, but no other problems appeared. After this time, he saw no need for further observation.

Carrie tells of the response to her healing. "A lot of people were very surprised and amazed. Even my mom, who wasn't a Christian, told me, 'Wow, God saved your life. You need to live for Him.' Two non-Christians I knew who were medical doctors had been following me and my condition, because they had been very concerned. They couldn't believe what had happened. One of them told me one day, 'You know, if I had not seen this with my own eyes, I wouldn't believe it.' But it *was* true, and soon after that, he became a Christian. I was so thankful. I think the experience and the witness that it was definitely helped him come to God."

Carrie thinks back over all she's gone through. "I think that God has been and still is very merciful with me. Extremely merciful. He loves me so much. With the first miracle that I had, He actually let me experience His concern, not just for my physical being, but my spiritual and emotional health first. I was brought to a place where I saw my spiritual need and was able to repent. If He had not shown me, I don't think I would ever have done that; I think I would still be a very arrogant person. But He took care of all my needs: physically, emotionally, and spiritually. Sometimes I ask God, 'Why are you so merciful with me? Who am I? I haven't done anything that's particularly good or holy or anything!' But God so unselfishly just poured out His love for me. And that has definitely transformed my whole life."

Carrie herself thanked God in the end for the struggle she went through with endometriosis. Though at the time it was extremely difficult and physically painful, the change it brought about in her and the richness of relationship with Christ that it brought her into were treasures she wouldn't trade for the world. And while the fear she felt about her kidneys and the surgeries they would require was certainly almost paralyzing at the time, the testimony of healing she now has and the people [who] have come to Christ because of it are results that Carrie and Tommy praise God for.

Reviving Dr. Luke

Largely as a result of their experience of healing, Tommy and Carrie have become heavily involved with The International Order of St.

Luke the Physician (OSL), an international ministry that brings the practice of healing into the church. Dr. Colin Campbell is the Canadian Director of OSL and first directed me to hear Tommie and Carrie's story. Below he tells about the group and his experience with them.

Q: What is the purpose of the Order of St. Luke's?

Colin: The purpose of St. Luke's (OSL) is to spread the knowledge of the type of healing that was done by Jesus in the New Testament stories, and as was carried out by the early Christian Church until about the year 300. So the basic purpose of OSL is to carry out the emotional, physical, and spiritual healing and make it available. OSL began in the 1920s through Anglican Archbishop William Temple, whose main objective was to get healing back into the mainline church. It then spread to America in 1936. The Order of St. Luke was formed by John Gaynor Banks and his wife, Ethel Banks.

Q: What kind of healings have you seen through your connection with the OSL?

Colin: I've really seen all. I've seen physical healings. I've seen mainly spiritual healings and what's called healing of memories. I'll give you one example that illustrates that aspect. A woman had come in and her husband had lost the sight in one eye and was losing it in the other. Her son was on drugs and she had an adolescent daughter [who] was reasonably normal, but had a lot of reasons for stress. So she came in asking for prayer.

I started praying for these things and nothing was happening. And then I stopped and I asked God, 'So, what am I supposed to be praying for?' And what I saw, was a baby girl in the hands of her father. And so He said, 'Ask her about her childhood.' So I said, 'Could you tell me about your childhood, specifically about your father?' And it turned out that her father had died when she was ten years old, and her mother had said, 'You mustn't grieve for your father. He wouldn't want you to. He'd want you to move on.' She hadn't been allowed to grieve for her father and ever since that time, apparently, she had been depressed in her adolescence. So I prayed for her to give herself permission to grieve. And she sobbed. The floor was wet. She sobbed for ten minutes.

The other is spiritual healing [occurs when] the person isn't living a Christian life at all. And they need to, in a classical term, need to be saved. [They] need to be born again.

Q: Why is healing (or the gift of healing) so important, that we should emphasize it?

Colin: The goal of Christian life, just to set a perspective, in my opinion, is spiritual transformation. The ultimate healing is a relationship with God in this life and beyond this life. The ultimate goal of life is to have abundant life, fullness of life that comes out of a relationship with God. It's a spiritual relationship, not a moral relationship, not an intellectual relationship, but a spiritual relationship [that] includes and is based on the emotions.

We're built in the image of God. That image is brought out in the emotional or spiritual life. The mind is drawn into the spirit to kind of form categories [that's] completely scientific. Science is not based on the mind or philosophy; it's based on experience and so on. So that way of knowing is central to both, I would think.

Let's take the issue of healing. My view of that is, of course, Jesus healed instantly. It wasn't a process; He healed instantly. While spiritual transformation is a process, it's something we go through. My way of putting this together is that spiritual transformation is the goal that only happens if we are open to the experience. You know the old William Holman Hunt image of Jesus knocking at the door, and the handle is on the inside because we must open the door? The people in the Bible were desperate for healing so the door was open, so Jesus could go in because He had the faith and power to heal and people were healed instantly. He didn't heal the rich young ruler that way, though, because that wasn't the need of the person had. The rich young ruler was bound by possessions. He couldn't open the door and went away very sad.

I see healing in that kind of perspective. The conditions need to be that it has to be the greatest need that the person has. Second, they must be open to a healing. And if the greatest need is not that, there's some spiritual element—lack of forgiveness for people, or false goals and so on—if that's a greater need, then that's what the Holy Spirit is going to target. I guess to answer your question, why healing? Well it depends on what you mean.

To limit healing to simply good behaviour and good values and ignore spiritual healing and deliverance—I think we've probably gone that way. And that perspective needs to be corrected.

Q: Why did healing fall out of favour in the church?

Colin: I think there are a couple of reasons. One is historical—the way the Church developed. And the other is scientific, the western culture in which we live. I can speak to both of those.

If we take the Church issue first, there was the Gnostic controversy throughout the first few centuries of Christianity. And Irenaeus formalized the church in order to deal with the Gnostic heresy. He formalized it in two ways. One: He expanded the role of the Bishops, he centralized the authority of the church. Things were not allowed to happen without permission of ecclesiastical authority figures. [Two]: Prayer and Christian worship [were] formalized as a liturgy. These were two things, ritualizing and formalizing, and eliminating the place for healing.

And what's [ironic] is Irenaeus did heal. It was documented that he raised someone from the dead. He carried on the tradition of healing, but was determined to stamp out Gnosticism, since he was against the Gnostic heresies. Healing didn't completely disappear, but it was centralized [on] a formalized liturgy around the Mass. Then people's healings were centralized around saints and relics.

And when we fast-forward to the Reformation, healing was associated with Catholicism in the mind of the Reformers, and was regarded as a superstition since it was centred on the worship of relics. The process of formalizing the liturgy was then transferred to a worship that was centred on the Word. And it became a more cerebral activity, where you studied the Scriptures to find out the will of God and the direction of God. And that produced a liberal reaction [through which] exegesis and hermeneutics became the way the clergy were trained. So that's one line of development.

The other line of development began with [Isaac] Newton, of course—[when] Newton said that everything is made up of particles in motion. And his laws of motion could describe why things happen, including why bodies were healed. And so it gave us Western medicine based on chemistry, which is based on Newton's laws.

Now what's significant for me as a physicist is that Newton's laws are wrong. They work because they have a symbolism that corresponds to reality as a sort of metaphor, if you like, that Newton discovered, that replicates the way things take place. But it isn't in fact real, because there are no particles. There's only energy [that] appears in the form of waves. It's a very recent discovery, which, of course, is quite compatible with a spiritual view of the world. If the spiritual view of the world underlies the material description (which it does, in fact), then healing and so on is perfectly possible and reconcilable with modern science.

I think the Church needs this reminder that healing is available to us. It needs a faith that matters in a whole new way. The Church does a good job of providing social services...a good job at providing community and identity. I think groups that promote healing are the missing piece that the Church should take seriously and begin to work with.

To conclude, from Dr. Colin Campbell, the Order of St. Luke's objectives are:

- "Promoting the restoration of the Apostolic practice of healing as taught and demonstrated by Jesus Christ;
- promoting a sound pastoral and counseling ministry;
- promoting the practice of holding healing services in every church; and
- developing local chapters to promote healing missions, workshops and prayer groups in their area."

Here are the Order of St. Luke's guidelines:

- "God uses many agencies for healing: some are spiritual such as prayer, love, faith, anointing with oil, and the laying on of hands;
- some are medical such as medicine, surgery, and psychology.
- These agencies should be supportive of one another.
- God's desire for us is wholeness and health.
- Christian healing is accomplished through faith in Christ and through subjecting one's entire life to the scrutiny and counsel of God.
- We believe Jesus Christ is alive today and still possesses all power on earth as in Heaven."

To learn more: https://orderofstluke.org/ru/about/become-part-of-the-osl-community.html

For a similar approach in a Catholic healing ministry: https://www.christianhealingmin.org/index.php/about-chm

Chapter 11

THE SCIENCE OF SPIRITUALITY AND HEALING

I praise you because I am fearfully and wonderfully
made; your works are wonderful, I know that full well.
—PSALM 139:14

Scientific studies are establishing spirituality as a clinically relevant
and beneficial factor when it comes to maintaining and restoring
health. However, as old ideas that regard the body and mind as mu-
tually exclusive stubbornly continue, spirituality still remains to be
neglected and mishandled in much of the published research found
in the traditional health and mental health literature.[65]

Our hope is, as such research continues, this will change. In
this chapter, we will look at some of the research on spirituality and
health as published by those who are engaged in it.

The Healing Power of Faith

Dr. Harold Koenig is Associate Professor of Psychiatry and Behavioral
Sciences and Assistant Professor of Medicine at Duke University Medical Center in North Carolina, as well as the Director of Duke University's Center for Spirituality, Theology and Health. He describes the
latter as "the world's first major research facility to comprehensively

study the impact of people's religious life on their physical and emotional health.[66]

He began his medical career as an orderly and nurse. He credits this beginning with his interest in the healing power of faith, because he had learned to listen to his patients. It was through listening to his patients' stories that he began to wonder about the relationship between their faith and their healing.

His first study involved looking at the relationship between religious belief and practice and death anxiety among several hundred elderly people attending senior lunch programs. The results were significant: 10.3 percent of the deeply religious people experienced death anxiety compared to twenty-five percent of the less religious. These early findings encouraged him to proceed with further research.[67]

Dr. Koenig makes an important distinction between "intrinsic" and "extrinsic" religiosity in his research. People with "intrinsic" faith not only practice their faith personally and corporately, but also live their everyday lives out of that faith. They are people who have a personal relationship with God, go to church at least once a week, pray and read their Bible regularly, and are involved in their faith community. People with "extrinsic" faith tend to go to church less often, pray or read their Bible less often, and are more likely to attend church for social, status, or political reasons.[68] While people with "extrinsic" faith reap some benefit, it is the people with "intrinsic" faith who benefit much more from the healing power of faith.

Among the findings of The Duke Center's research studies, Dr. Koenig has discovered that:[69]

- People who regularly attend church, pray individually, and read the Bible have significantly lower diastolic blood pressure than the less religious. Those with the lowest blood pressure both attend church and pray or study the Bible often.

- People who attend church regularly are hospitalized much less often than people who never or rarely participate in religious services.

- People with strong religious faith are less likely to suffer depression from stressful life events, and if they do, they are more likely to recover from depression than those who are less religious.

- The deeper a person's religious faith, the less likely he or she is to be crippled by depression during and after hospitalization for physical illness.

- Religious people have healthier lifestyles. They tend to avoid alcohol and drug abuse, risky sexual behaviour, and other unhealthy habits.

- Elderly people with a deep, personal ("intrinsic") religious faith have a stronger sense of wellbeing and life satisfaction than their less religious peers. This may be due in part to the stable marriages and strong families religious people tend to build.

- People with strong faith who suffer from physical illness have significantly better health outcomes than less religious people.

- People who attend religious services regularly have stronger immune systems than their less religious counterparts.

- Religious people live longer, physically healthier. Religious faith appears to protect the elderly from the two major afflictions of later life, cardiovascular disease, and cancer.

The Faith Factor

It came as no surprise to Dr. Dale Matthews, a specialist in internal medicine and former faculty member at Yale and other universities, when numerous scientific studies demonstrated that religious faith and commitment have a positive impact on health and healing. He had often made that observation during the years of practicing as a physician. In fact, he learned on his first day of medical school what kind of doctor he did not want to become. He had gone into medicine hoping to learn and practice compassionate, person-centred doctoring, yet here he "ran headlong into a different world, one where the biochemistry of molecules was valued more highly than the pain of human beings."[70]

In his book, *The Faith Factor*, which he co-wrote with Connie Clark, Matthews writes that:

> The clinical emergence of 'the faith factor' in medicine is an unexpected development for those of us trained in Western medical schools. For some of my colleagues, the idea of including spirituality in clinical care comes as a challenge, if not an outright shock. For me, however, the need to address patients' spiritual needs was not a surprise; rather it grew naturally out of my deep-seated commitment to the doctor-patient relationship.[71]

Matthews does not hesitate to address spiritual issues with his patients and demonstrates this in his book with many personal anecdotes. He suggests that to do so would be to neglect or ignore prescribing a healing remedy that may very well be the key to their wholeness and healing. He believes that, given the scientific evidence emerging today about religious involvement and health, "doctors who want to help other human beings who suffer, doctors who want to be healers of whole persons, have an obligation to address the spiritual lives of their patients."[72] He suggests that doctors could, from a strictly scientific point of view, recommend religious involvement to their patients to help improve their chances of being able to:[73]

- Stay healthy and avoid life-threatening and disabling diseases like cancer and heart disease.
- Recover faster and with fewer complications if they do develop a serious illness.
- Live longer.
- Encounter life-threatening and terminal illnesses with greater peacefulness and less pain.
- Avoid mental illnesses like depression and anxiety, and cope more effectively with stress.
- Steer clear of problems with alcohol, drugs, and tobacco.
- Enjoy a happier marriage and family life.
- Find a greater sense of meaning and purpose in life.

Dr. Matthews makes the distinction between spirituality and religion, and their impact when they are intricately connected:

> ...'spirituality' connotes an individual's private search for meaning and connection, particularly his or her relationship with God, 'religion' suggests the individual's adherence to an organized set of beliefs and practices endorsed by a community of fellow believers. One can be religious and spiritual; in fact, the evidence points to this combination as the ideal for enhancing health and well-being.[74]

Like Koenig, Matthews also recognizes "intrinsic" and "extrinsic" religiosity. A healthy, life-giving religion would include "spirituality" practices in the context of a person's "religion."

Matthews identifies twelve essential remedies for various aspects of life where human beings need wholeness and healing. In one part of his book, he looks at them from a medical perspective; in another section, he shows how each of these components form part of religious worship services. By participating in worship, each of these "remedies" can help us in becoming whole persons. These remedies include: equanimity, temperance, beauty, adoration, renewal, community, unity, ritual, meaning, trust, transcendence, and love. Tending to a balanced diet of each of these aspects in life and worship has been shown scientifically to enhance health and wholeness.

God, Faith, and Health

Epidemiology is the science of looking at the various factors that make people sick or help them to remain healthy. Several scientists have now included factors such as membership in religious communities, faith, or religious practices in their calculations.[75] Among these is Dr. Jeff Levin, epidemiologist and Professor of Epidemiology and Population Health, Professor of Medical Humanities, and Director of the Program on Religion and Population Health at Baylor Institute for Studies of Religion.

In the many scientific studies he has investigated, as well as in research studies he himself has conducted with colleagues in his field, he has found that the spirituality-healing connection is, indeed, significant for religious people of all faiths. He has formulated seven principles as the result of his research:

Principle One: Religious affiliation and membership benefit health by promoting healthy behavior and lifestyles.

Most religions endorse the idea that we ought to take care of our bodies and not act in ways that are reckless and endanger our lives, in line with the biblical idea that *"your body is a temple of the Holy Spirit within you, [whom] you have from God,"* (1 Corinthians 6:19, ESV).[76] The degree to which religious affiliation and membership benefit health and wellbeing depends on a faith community's emphasis on behavioural demands and the degree to which adherents follow them.[77]

Principle Two: Regular religious fellowship benefits health by offering support that buffers the effects of stress and isolation.

Religious attendance is a social behaviour, one not practiced in isolation, but rather in the company of other fellow believers. When we worship, we are with other people, sharing a common purpose. Being part of a faith community offers a theological worldview that makes sense out of a chaotic world, and gives us a sense of connection to a benevolent "Divine Other." It also increases our access to people who can help when we are in need. In addition to the community gathered for worship there are many other opportunities to enjoy regular fellowship in smaller groups for prayer, Bible study, and meditation.[78]

Principle Three: Participation in worship and prayer benefits health through the physiological effects of positive emotions.

Public worship with others, ideally, elicits feelings of interpersonal trust, mutuality, and intimacy. Worship rituals, such as prayer, give structure and context to our encounters with God. Worship activates what psychologists call "attachment" processes that connect people both to one another and to God, especially if their image of God is that of a loving heavenly Father.[79]

Through a recent study, Levin discovered that feeling love for or feeling loved by God was associated with greater self-esteem, higher levels of self-efficacy or sense of mastery, less depression, less physical disability, and greater self-rated health. A principle means of experiencing positive emotions, especially feelings of love and forgiveness, is by religious worship and prayer, both public and private.[80] Levin suggests that such emotional responses may be powerful sources of health and healing through:

> ...bolstering our resistance to disease and strengthening the body's immunity and ability to maintain a healthy homeostasis or balance, the positive emotions resulting from religious worship can help us to negotiate and overcome the stresses of daily life.[81]

Keeping the lines of communication open with God is among the healthiest things we can do. Our relationship with God, in turn, influences how we get along with others, how we respond to stress, how we deal with daily events, and how we feel about ourselves.[82]

Principle Four: Religious beliefs benefit health by their similarity to health-promoting beliefs and personality styles.

For some people, religious rituals, such as public worship or private prayer, are welcome interludes, providing moments of respite in our hectic lives.

These brief connections to the eternal bring peace, contentment, and health and wellbeing and may be a source of strength, sustenance, and healing. For others, religious practice is not just a joyful interruption in an otherwise-secular life. Rather, it reflects a spiritual worldview or belief system that permeates all aspects of life, influencing every dimension of life. It is the central and defining feature of their entire personality. The one is doing religion, the other is being religious, and evidence appears to indicate that being religious is beneficial for health and overall wellbeing.[83]

Principle Five: Simple faith benefits health by leading to thoughts of hope, optimism, and positive expectation.

Longitudinal studies have shown that people who rated themselves as more religious had greater life satisfaction and happiness, as well as fewer symptoms of depression. Being or feeling religious, not just practicing religion, has protective effects that last far into the future.[84] Faith, through its provision of hope and positive expectations, is epidemiologically significant.[85] Levin suggests that faith deserves a place at the table in discussions of factors known to prevent illness and promote health and wellbeing alongside other considerations. When we exclude faith from scientific discussions of the determinants of health, we arbitrarily rule out a potentially powerful ally in reducing distress and promoting health.[86]

For the above five principles, there is much evidence that private spiritual expression and public religious participation benefit a person's health. Levin believes that through behavioural, social, and psychological functions, religion and spirituality alleviate distress and promote wellbeing, both physically and emotionally. He calls these aspects "active ingredients," and believes these are now well-accepted by medical science. There is now growing evidence to show that religion also influences our health through other pathways, the discovery of which is at the cutting edge of science and still quite controversial.[87] The following two principles fit into this category and are now being explored, by Levin and others, to determine their impact on health and healing.

Principle Six: Mystical experiences benefit health by activating a healing bioenergy or life force or altered state of consciousness.

Levin differentiates between "exoteric" religion—that is, faith exercised in the context of a faith community, and "esoteric" religion, an inner spirituality not practiced in a religious community. The more typical expression of the latter type of spirituality is daily meditation or incorporation of contemplative elements into traditional rituals, rather than weekly church attendance. Such activities often result in experiencing transcendent or mystical states, altered states of consciousness, and a sense of union or connection with God or the divine.[88]

Levin observes that mystical experiences tend to be viewed with "varying degrees of apprehension among traditionally religious people."[89] Yet such experiences are surprisingly common among people practicing exoteric as well as esoteric religion.[90] A study of 200 Christians found that mystical experiences led to feelings of oneness, connection, and lasting beneficial psychological changes. An experience that "resonates within the experiencer as making sense, containing great meaning, and offering direction or redirection to one's life can be a powerful source of psychological growth."[91] However, Levin cautions that for such experiences to have positive, healing outcomes, people should seek solid grounding in their faith tradition that "can frame, interpret, and make sense of such things."[92]

Findings suggest that certain types of mystical experiences are associated with feelings of wellbeing, especially when such experiences were associated with greater "meaning in life," finding purpose and satisfaction in one's life. As in other research, this was associated with greater health.[93]

Principle Seven: Absent prayer for others is capable of healing by paranormal means or by divine intervention.

Levin suggests there are two possible sources of answered prayers. One is "naturalistic," where the healing response originates from within nature. The other he terms "supernatural," where people are healed because God hears and responds to their prayers.

That's not to say that God can't also heal through the natural laws of the universe. It's the latter understanding of prayer, that God hears and heals, he suggests, that is the cornerstone of many of the world's faith traditions. Levin believes that science, by definition, will never be able to prove the existence of supernatural healing, nor can it disprove it.[94]

Chapter 12

TAKING ACTION ON BELIEF IN HEALING FAITH

I rise before dawn and cry for help; I have put my hope
in your word. My eyes stay open through the watches
of the night, that I may meditate on your promises.
—PSALM 119:147–148

In recent years, a great number of books, magazine and newspaper articles, and TV documentaries have tackled the issue of spirituality and healing and the healing power of prayer. Religious people have always prayed and believed that faith and prayer make a difference. However, now, as we have seen, numerous scientific studies are demonstrating that, indeed, prayer and spiritual practices can—and do—make a difference in healing and wholeness.

Prayer

There is nothing uniquely Christian about prayer. There is something inherent in the human spirit, when threatened by the unknown, that cries out to whatever unseen powers there may be that appear to control the universe. Prayer arises from the human sense of the transcendent, a power beyond what we can see or touch.[95] While there is something beautiful about this, pointing to the innate human knowledge that there is something beyond what is seen, we should be careful to note that not all forms of prayer are equal.

Howard L. Rice, Professor of Ministry and Chaplain Emeritus at San Francisco Theological Seminary identifies two main types of prayer. The first one is the universal crying out to God in time of need; the second is our willing abandonment of self to God's will. He compares the two:

> There is a radical difference between prayer as getting God to do our bidding and prayer as increased self-understanding and changing us to conform more nearly to God's will. If the one form of prayer is 'universal' and 'natural,' the other form of prayer is 'God-centered' and 'relational.' The purpose of the first is to get something and the purpose of the second is to become something.[96]

Rice suggests some guidelines to remember that can help us to see prayer as relationship with God more than as pleading for what we want: 1) Prayer is both corporate and personal; 2) Prayer is both spontaneous and disciplined; 3) Prayer is an affair of the mind and the heart; and 4) We need to pray as both speaker and hearer.[97]

For a long time, we have lived with a worldview that understands nature as operating according to fixed laws. Such a view of nature limits God, and leads to the belief that prayer can't make any difference. People often lack trust that God can change the way things are. It seems pointless to pray when changes can only come about by our own accomplishments. Consequently, Rice posits, the chief hindrances to prayer in the twentieth century are:

> ...distorted images of God which cause us to avoid a close companionship with God and distorted images of ourselves

which cause us to seek to prove our own self-sufficiency by trying to go it alone. A recovery of a Christological focus for our image of God and a recovery of a sense of our need for God in order for us to be fully human are both a deep part of our Reformed heritage.[98]

Numerous scientific studies have been undertaken to determine the effectiveness of prayer. One of the earliest and most famous studies on this subject to become publicized was the 1988 study by American cardiologist, Dr. Randolph C. Byrd. It took place in the coronary-care unit of the San Francisco General Hospital. The study included 393 patients who were randomly assigned to two groups. One group of 192 patients were prayed for daily, until their discharge, by Christians from around the country, knowing them only by name and clinical status. The other 201 patients, the control group, did not receive this experimental prayer. Participants knew of the study, but did not know to which group they belonged.

In each area of measurement, the prayed-for group did considerably better. Among the control group, there were twenty who had episodes of congestive heart failure compared to eight among the prayed-for group. The use of diuretics was a third less in the prayed-for group. Episodes of cardiopulmonary arrest were fourteen to three, episodes of pneumonia thirteen to three, use of antibiotics seventeen to three, favouring those who were prayed for. Of the control group, twelve required intubation, while none of the prayed-for group did.[99]

In commenting on Dr. Byrd's study, Sister Barbara Fiand, in *Prayer and the Quest for Healing*, suggests that "prayer resonance" is both physically and spiritually effective. By "prayer resonance," she means "the belief in our interconnectedness on a deeper level of consciousness which allows us to send 'prayer resonance' or healing power to one another over a great distance."[100]

She relates an experiment on how this type of prayer works:

A group of twenty-eight people wanting to experiment with this concept chose a high-crime area of a large U.S. city, praying and meditating six nights in a row for one hour. Computerized police statistics recorded a drop in the crime rate of twenty-nine percent below the crime rate of the remainder of the city. When the experiment was repeated several weeks later, similar results were recorded.[101]

The question arises as to how prayers are answered, whether by our interconnectedness and caring in sending healing power to another even over a great distance or through God's answer to our prayers. This is the same question Levin dealt with under his Principle Seven.

John Polkinghorne, a well-known theoretical physicist and theologian, would agree on the interconnectedness of everything. He believes that "we have power to act in the world and that God also has retained power to act in the world."[102] He suggests that in prayer, we are seeking to align those two actions as closely as possible. If we are open and prepared to offer ourselves and collaborate with God, our attitude will have consequences not only for ourselves but also for other people, because everything is linked together in the world. Knowing that "helps to explain why the praying of a lot of people for the same thing can achieve remarkable effects."[103]

Physician and author Dr. Larry Dossey thought he had left prayer far back in his past until he read of a single scientific study supporting the healing power of prayer. As a doctor, he felt the need to investigate this, not expecting to find much support for the idea. Much to his surprise, he discovered it was not the only study; in fact, there were hundreds. He was especially surprised that this was not common knowledge among scientifically trained physicians. But then he came to realize that "a body of knowledge that does not fit with prevailing ideas can be ignored as if it does not exist, no matter how scientifically valid it may be."[104]

Dossey also recognized he had to do something with that knowledge now that he could no longer deny it. He has done much more than using it only in his medical practice. Like Matthews, he came to the place where he decided that "not to employ prayer with my patients was the equivalent of deliberately withholding a potent drug or surgical procedure."[105]

He has also written a number of books on the efficacy of prayer and cites the results of many scientific studies which show the healing power of prayer not only for human beings but also for animals, plants, and cells. The effectiveness of prayer is not altered by distance. He suggests that if he had to single out one quality that correlates with effective prayer in the scientific studies, it would be love, or compassion, or empathy; in other words, you have to *care*.[106]

Other Faith Practices

In addition to prayer, there are several other faith practices that have also proven to promote healing for those who practice them. Different authors focus on different practices that form part of a healthy spirituality; however, they appear to be in agreement with one another. We will look at several of the faith practices considered beneficial to healing.

Dr. Dale Matthew identifies three essential aspects of a healthy, life-enhancing spirituality that have been shown scientifically to make a significant difference. He deals in some length with each one in *The Faith Factor*. They include 1) Regular private and communal prayer; 2) Reading, meditating, and studying the riches of the Scriptures; and 3) Being an active member of a loving spiritual community.

Ronald Rolheiser, president of the Oblate School of Theology in San Antonio, Texas, identifies what he calls four essential, non-negotiable pillars that he believes undergird any healthy Christian spirituality and practice.

They are: a) Private prayer and private morality; b) Social justice; c) Mellowness of heart and spirit; and d) Community as a constitutive element of true worship. Rolheiser emphasizes the necessity of balance among these four essentials and relates several scenarios to show what happens when one aspect is missing. Perhaps the essential that may be least self-evident is "mellowness of heart and spirit," which, he suggests, has to do with gratitude. We can do all the right things for the wrong reasons—for instance, out of anger, guilt, grandiosity, or self-interest. Like the older brother of the prodigal son, we can be faithful in our service and yet bitter of heart.[107]

Christian theologian, professor and author Richard Foster found himself wondering if there wasn't something more and began searching the tradition more broadly.

He discovered many treasures, which he explores in detail in his *Celebration of Discipline: The Path to Spiritual Growth*, under three main headings: 1) The inward disciplines, including meditation, prayer, fasting, and study; 2) The outward disciplines of simplicity, solitude, submission, and service; and 3) The corporate disciplines of confession, worship, guidance, and celebration.[108]

All the above authors would agree that not only are these faith practices essential aspects of a healthy spirituality, but they would also affirm their potential to be a part of a healthy lifestyle and in restoring wholeness and healing in body, mind, and spirit.

Believing in Healing Today

For centuries, the spiritual and religious beliefs of people, lived out in their daily lives, along with folk remedies, were all that people had for their healing. In the Bible, both the Old and New Testaments speak of physicians, but they had little to offer in terms of alleviating pain and suffering and restoring health and wholeness.

While people of the Christian faith have always prayed for themselves and others in the face of illness, most still tend to put their trust for health and healing in their physician, increasingly so as medicine has found the answer to many of our diseases. Perhaps it was at the point when people realized that science and medicine have their limitations that they began to consider alternative ways of healing. It has also become apparent that science and medicine, while offering us many benefits, have focused too much on the human body at the expense of the whole human person.

As we have seen, those who recognized this limitation in the early stages of the development of medical research were hesitant to voice their hunches. There appears to be a correlation between the yearning for wholeness we see, the re-emergence of healing ministries in mainline churches, and the scientific studies showing that prayer and other faith practices are having a profound effect on healing. Professor Polkinghorne believes that:

> ...logically there isn't a contradiction between science and religion because they are both trying to find the truth through motivated belief. They are, of course, looking at different aspects of the truth. Science is looking at an impersonal world that it can put to the test. Religion is looking at a personal and a transpersonal world involving God, where testing has to give way to trusting.[109]

For most Christians, it's not either medicine or divine healing in response to prayer. Christians appreciate and expect to be prayed for. They are grateful whether healing comes instantaneously, through a doctor's skill, or the body's own healing system; all are the gift of God. Ultimately, we believe that all healing is from God who has made us.

The Church is once again believing that it's able to practice a healing ministry drawing on the same power that Jesus drew on in his earthly ministry. Prayer still forms the basis of the ministry of healing. As people of faith, we have many resources to live healthy, holistic lives, such as our faith that is lived out in the context of a faith community, which many scientific studies affirm. In addition to this, we may take advantage of the healing remedies administered through medical science. These are gifts from a compassionate and loving God, from whom all healing comes.

Chapter 13

A JOURNEY OF FULL RESTORATION

Therefore, if anyone is in Christ, the new creation has
come: The old has gone, the new is here!
—2 CORINTHIANS 5:17

Life had never been easy for Rebecca. Her father wasn't around
when she was a child. She had suffered multiple cases of abuse.
To make matters worse, resources were spread thin on her remote
Northern Quebec Reserve, and health issues were rampant. She was
headed for a life of emotional, mental, and physical health issues—
that is, until God intervened.

Rebecca was affected by the faith of Quebec Cree businessman
and chief, Billy Diamond. "I was just curious about his ministry,
though I didn't want to go at first, not until a friend invited me. But
the way he expressed God was so real—the message was about His
Father heart and the healing of our hearts; I didn't know God could
be my Father!"

She goes on, detailing the impact Billy had in her life and in her
community. "God used [Billy Diamond] to be a spiritual father to
me and to help me to forgive my biological father. He did a lot. He
brought hope. Before, I had no hope, I felt I had no life. I didn't know

I was able to enjoy life again. I didn't know God could be so real, such a loving Father, and that Jesus could be more than a friend."

She explains more of the changes she's seen in herself. "Before I was so shy, I didn't have any confidence, I didn't believe in myself, I couldn't speak. But [Billy] believed in me, and he just loved me. I felt safe with him."

"God healed me a lot, from all kinds of abuse and situations [in which] I had to extend a lot of grace to people," she continues. "I even had to extend a lot of grace and a lot of forgiveness to myself for the things I did in my past. Now, I don't have to condemn myself; even if I fail, the best part is that He still loves me."

Tackling Rebecca's past and emotional health was the first step and is an ongoing one. Through journaling and spending many hours in intimate conversation with God, she is able to hold on to truth and stay free of all shame and pain from her past. But her physical health was still yet to be addressed.

An intense work schedule began worsening Rebecca's weight problem and her diabetes along with it. When several adults in their thirties and forties died suddenly from various health problems in Rebecca's community, she woke up to the urgency of addressing her own wellbeing. This coincided with a friend's suggestion that she come to study at a school of ministry in Toronto, where she was also told there was better access to resources for First Nations people.

Upon coming to Toronto, she was soon connected with Anishnawbe Health Toronto. "They had a diabetes team and a nutritionist and physiotherapist I could see regularly. Back home, they would just fly in and you had to wait on the list, so it took a while to be seen for physiotherapy," she explains. "Then, with the nutritionist, I was challenged to write down the foods that were really controlling me. In the beginning, it was hard, especially on weekends, which was my time for comfort food. But slowly, I had to say, 'I can do this.' Sometimes I would fail, but when I did, I tried not to be too harsh with myself. I would say, 'Okay, yesterday I failed, but today it's a new day. What can I do? What do I do to learn from this?'"

Rebecca went on to join an AquaFit class, then later started exercising with a trainer, slowly increasing the amount of cardio training she could do. With discipline and perseverance, Rebecca went on to lose about sixty pounds.

"In the beginning, I didn't believe I could do it," Rebecca says. "I never thought I would be off insulin, but I've been off over two years now. And, as for the pills, now I'm just taking vitamins, and I have only one medication left."

Rebecca's journey has been slow, but it's also been steady. God has addressed one area of her life at a time, bringing her to a place of holistic health. Rebecca affirms, "I want to be healthy for life. I know though that it's a lifetime commitment. It's every day."

Her assurance that God is deserving of all the praise for her recovery and growth is solid. "I do believe God can heal people. He's not just a God who sits up there; He's a God of today, He's a God of the past, and He's the God of future. I truly believe God can restore anybody. When I think about my life now, it is all thanks to the work of God—both where I'm at today, and where I'm going to be in the future."

The good news is that Christ came to redeem and restore *all* that was broken. There is no nook or cranny that brokenness invaded that He cannot take back under the victory of His cross. The diversity of characters that Jesus recruited as His followers demonstrates this.

Luke 19:1–10 tells the story of Zacchaeus, a greedy traitor, exiled from his community for selling out to the Roman authorities and using his position to cheat his own countrymen out of their hard-earned money. But Jesus cured him of his greed and even humbled him into giving back all that he had wrongfully taken.

The woman at the well was an outcast, as well. She had to draw water in the middle of the day when all the other women would have done so long before, when the sun was cooler. Whether she was a serial victim or there was something else going on, she had had many husbands, had lost them all and now lived with a man to whom she was not married. But after her encounter with Jesus, she ran into the centre of town to boldly proclaim that she had met the Messiah. Due to her testimony, many people sought Him out and believed.

Peter was impulsive, acting and speaking first, then thinking later. But he also suffered from a great fear of man. In the hours before Christ's crucifixion, he denied he knew him. Later, when he was a leader of the new Christian Church, he began snobbishly excluding himself from the company of Gentiles in order to impress the prominent Jewish Christians in the group.

With what was a seemingly lifelong struggle, when Peter was confronted about his shortfall, he repented, and church tradition holds that he was eventually crucified upside down for his faith, suggesting that he had overcome his fear of man and was finally standing strong for what he believed in, even if that meant crucifixion.

In all three cases, the people suffered from a past or shortcoming that likely caused them shame. They might have felt hopeless, might have felt that this thorn was so much a part of their identity that there was no hope of being free of it, or being the kind of person they would be proud of. But Christ proved them wrong.

One by one, either instantly or in a process over time, all were made free and new again. While we often talk about Jesus bearing our *sins* on the cross, Isaiah 53:4 states that, *"Surely he has borne our griefs and carried our sorrows; yet we esteemed him stricken, smitten by God, and afflicted"* (ESV). Not only has Christ picked up and defeated our sin, He has also borne our griefs and our sorrows. Our griefs and sorrows may be related to sins we've committed, or they may be tied to sins committed against us, or they may be tied to seemingly random circumstances that aren't anyone's fault at all. Whatever it is that is burdening us, it is inherently tied to brokenness, and because of this, it belongs to the realm of what has been defeated and reclaimed by Christ as His own.

With the cross, Jesus accomplished healing for our past, if we are willing to step into it. With the Holy Spirit, He promises a plan of growth for the future. The result of the Holy Spirit in our lives is the development of "...*love, joy, peace, patience, kindness, goodness, faithfulness, gentleness, self-control*" (Galatians 5:22–23, ESV).

With the Holy Spirit's sanctifying power, He will surgically remove the spiritual infections that are no longer fitting for our lives. This may be our impatience, hatefulness, envy, cowardice, manipulative selfishness, or something else entirely. In their place, He will put characteristics of Himself, and by doing so, will make us more into our true selves, the ones created in His image finally becoming who they were intended to be.

Chapter 14

BACK FROM A HEART ATTACK

Again, truly I tell you that if two of you on earth agree
about anything they ask for, it will be done for them by
my Father in heaven. For where two or three gather in
my name, there am I with them.
—MATTHEW 18:19–20

Bev and Bill Beck were married at both twenty-four years old, and for the next forty-eight years, their lives were blessed with children, a secure home, a rich church community life, travel, and togetherness. But the years were not entirely without their trials. Bill, in particular, had experienced troubles with his heart. Some chest pain when he was fifty resulted in a quadruple bypass surgery, and at sixty-five years, he had a mild heart attack while on vacation with his wife in Israel. But at seventy-two, Bill suffered a complete cardiac arrest.

"I can remember him at the bedroom door. He said, 'I'll see you later'," Bev says, thinking back on the day. "He was taking a bit longer than usual to come back home. Then I got the phone call. They said, 'Is this Mrs. Beck?' and I said, 'Yes.' And they said, 'Bill Beck is dead.'"

Bev was numb and in shock. Her pastor came over immediately, and together they headed to the hospital. They found out that, after numerous attempts with the defibrillator paddles, the medical personnel were finally able to get a heartbeat. Bill wasn't dead, but the situation was very bleak. Not only was there the obvious heart issue, but Bill had fallen very hard with the attack, and there was concern about his brain. Bev was at the hospital until 4:00 in the morning, waiting for any changes or signs of hope. None came.

"My kids told me I acted like I was numb. I was trying to take everything in, and I—I was concerned how I was going to be alone," says Bev, welling up with emotion. "That was the biggest thing. I knew he was happy, I knew where he was going. He had told me he was okay to go when God would take him. I had real peace about that, but he left me, and what was I going to do? He's my soulmate.

"But I also knew that God is in control, and He'll provide. He'll help me. He'll get me through it."

A Family Together in Prayer

Bev's daughter, a registered nurse, came the next day and moved in with Bev. She would stay for the whole ordeal, and along with the rest of family, there was plenty of support available for Bev.

Still, it wasn't easy for any of them. For ten days, they sat through various attempts to revive Bill in some way or another. The family would pray together through all of it, with Bev's daughter helping to explain what was happening medically. Finally, the doctors met with the family alone, and told them that there was nothing more they could do. They decided together to give Bill three more days, and then they would "pull the plug," the tough medical choice of withdrawing nutritional and ventilation support from Bill's body.

On the thirteenth day, at 5:00 in the afternoon, the family gathered around Bill in his hospital room. "As a family we stood there, and each individual prayed and gave him to the Lord. It was a precious, precious time, I'll never forget it," Bev remembers. At the end of their time together, they agreed with the doctors to withdraw all medical treatment and hydration, and the doctors "pulled the plug" for end of life. No one knew how long it would take for him to fade out completely, but they didn't think it would be very long. Meanwhile, grandchildren back home continued to pray, certain their grandfather was returning home. The family went to the funeral parlour and started to make arrangements.

An Unexpected Turn

But then Bev got a call the next morning and heard the very last thing she expected to hear. One of her daughters had been singing to Bill, and he had responded by asking to her to keep singing. Later in the afternoon, their pastor also heard him speak.

Bill did not look well, and the fact that he wasn't fading as they all expected almost frightened the family; if he did go on living, what quality of life would he have? But day by day, Bill improved, slowly regaining his balance, mobility, and clarity of mind. Before long, he was released from the hospital.

"I wasn't the only one in shock," Bev says. "The nurses really didn't know what to do. They had never had [seen] that happen before, ever."

Bill's case was so exceptional, he became something of a hospital celebrity. "Several months later, my wife and I went to visit a friend at the [same] hospital," Bill says. "We walked to the information desk and the lady said warmly, 'Hello, Mr. Beck!' She told my wife, 'Everybody in the hospital knows your husband.'"

Bev had her husband back, their children had their father back, and Bill had a second chance at life. "I've been able to share my story with literally hundreds of people, and each time I remind people that God answered the prayers of an awful lot of people from around the world. Even my cardiologist admitted, 'You are a walking miracle!'" Bill laughs. "And that's exactly how I feel. God performed a miracle. Yes, He used medical personnel, but it was God who performed the miracle."

"I'm praying for you" and "Our prayers are with you," are two of the most common phrases a Christian will hear during times of public or personal struggle. Perhaps it's been said so often we don't feel the impact of the phrase anymore, or perhaps we've said it so many times ourselves without following it up with any real prayer action, that we suspect others do the same and don't feel the phrase has any real meaning. But to brush the phrase off as meaningless would be a mistake.

In Ephesians 6, Paul outlines the "Armour of God," the practices and tools we must utilize to fight off that which aims to derail our faith. After naming each piece of armour, Paul then gives the command to *"pray in the Spirit on all occasions with all kinds of prayers and requests"* (Ephesians 6:18).

Prayer, then, is seen as the action of a warrior, the primary strategy of spiritual soldiers fighting in battle. It is not a limp, passive, empty ritual, or merely an obligatory act of respect we present to God in honour of those we know going through hard times. It is our first line of attack against all that is not of God in the world. It becomes our most effective line of attack by appealing to the Heavenly Champion for His representation in the fight.

Singer Bethany Dillon, in her song, "Those Who Wait," sings the line, "You can do more in my waiting than in my doing I can do." But sometimes we can feel like we are not doing enough when we are "just praying." We feel like we should get out and do something practical that will make a difference *now*.

While it's good and commendable to serve one another in practical ways, to toss aside our prayer time exclusively in favour of acts of service would be a mistake. And it would be one precisely for the reason that Bethany sings about: If we thought of the very best and most powerful thing we are capable of doing, our power to positively affect the situation would still be laughably miniscule compared to the impact God is capable of with a blink of His eye. He can do more in our waiting and praying than we in our doing can do. Therefore, the best way of fighting for our loved ones is often to spend more time appealing to the One who has the power to do something big, instead of fussing about, often in vain, to muster up a miracle ourselves.

The reason some of us may be leery of this is because we're afraid God won't act, and then we'll feel like we've just wasted our time. But do you really think that if God has decided a person's fate, you have the power to change it by not praying and trying to fix things yourself instead? Do you really think you can pull a "fast one" on God when He's not looking?

In His Sermon on the Mount, Jesus tells us we *"cannot make one hair white or black"* (Matthew 5:36), and in the next chapter, He asks, *"Can any one of you by worrying add a single hour to your life?"* (Matthew 6:27). Therefore, there really is no point whatsoever in deluding ourselves into believing that we can make an impact on the situation outside the hands of God, and we'll do our loved ones far better if we submit ourselves to prayer and to serving practically under that submissive and prayerful attitude.

"But when you ask, you must believe and not doubt, because the one who doubts is like a wave of the sea, blown and tossed by the wind" (James 1:6)

So, in all things, let our first strategy be to pray, trusting God for His action and His goodness in all actions—even apparent inaction. We serve a God who loves us, who delights in giving His children good gifts, and who does act on the prayers of His people. Bill Beck testifies that God responded to the prayers of hundreds of people when he essentially brought him back to life. God has responded to the prayers of fewer people in equally incredible ways, and when we believe in Him, there's no reason He can't act for us in the same way, too.

Chapter 15

A GUIDE FOR THE INNER WORK

And my God will meet all your needs according to the
riches of his glory in Christ Jesus. To our God and
Father be glory for ever and ever. Amen.
—PHILIPPIANS 4:19–20

Perhaps more than anything else, the neo-Pentecostal and charismatic movement has brought the enthusiastic practice of Scripture-based healing back into consciousness among followers of Jesus and curious observers. As a result, there has been more openness to, and an expectation of, the operation of the supernatural gifts of the Spirit, including healing. Increasingly, churches are having healing services and are experiencing God's healing power through the healing of body and soul.

New scientific evidence has shown that the miraculous is not so strange, after all, and the universe is not as rigid and predictable as was once thought and taught. There is much that we do not and cannot understand, much less explain. Many scientific studies have shown a close interrelationship between our bodies, minds, and spirits and have demonstrated the importance of our spiritual life and its practices for wholeness and health. We need not be ashamed or apologetic for our faith and our faith practices. They are good for us!

A Prayer to Belong

Maybe in picking up this book on health and spiritual life, you have concluded you are not as closely connected to God as you would like to be. That is a life-giving longing that is pulling at your mind, and I encourage you to take advantage of the benefits of belonging, not only to God, but also to a healing community of a local church.

It all begins with action in your mind, a willing prayer from your deepest intent that you can articulate in welcoming Jesus Christ into your whole life. A prayer that goes something like this:

Loving Jesus, I need You and I want You in all of my life. Into my thoughts, my actions, come in and be my Saviour. Jesus, I believe You sent a great correction into the human race by coming to earth, and dying for all sin and defeating it in Your resurrection.

I believe that You now reign in heaven over us all. I want to take away all my sin through Your death on the cross, and I receive the gift of Your forgiveness for everything I may have done wrong in my past, present, and future. Thank You for saving me. Teach me to hear Your voice, to walk in Your steps.

Amen.

Don't Ignore the Holy Spirit

God is so immense that His qualities are contained in the Trinity Being of Jesus, Father God, and Holy Spirit. The teaching and practice of being in constant relationship with the Holy Spirit, which enters into us upon claiming Jesus as our Lord, is an essential companion for life with God and a daily interaction.

A former mentor of mine, Rev. David Mainse, a Pentecostal pastor and founder of Crossroads Christian Communications who passed away in 2017, liked to say that how we respond to the Holy Spirit has much to do with our temperament. He'd tell me that just as an introvert will quietly mutter when receiving a shock from an electric socket, the same shock will elicit a shout and jump from an extrovert. Apply that to how people respond to the Holy Spirit, David told me, and you'll start to understand the mystery of the Holy Spirit.

I try to remember to pray daily to be filled with the Holy Spirit, to be in a listening posture for God's voice through the Holy Spirit, and to be responsive to obey and act on God's Spirit speaking into mine. It's a mystery how the Holy Spirit guides and moves among us, but it's as real as it is mysterious. In my own work as a journalist, this constant evidence of the Holy Spirit at work in people's lives is what drew me from news reporting as a journalist into Christian journalism. The stories of God "speaking" to people and the actions they did as a result, were just too irrefutable to ignore.

In 1988, while a young mom on a maternity leave from regular journalism, I was reading a daily newspaper and stirred by the absence of any stories about God in the news. I had a prayer that day, "God, let me impact the media for you..."

Proof of Answered Prayer

God has engaged that prayer through the Holy Spirit more than I could ever have imagined. Now, in 2018, that prayer has taken me to service as a CEO, leading Canada's largest Christian media outlet and Canada's most-watched religious TV Station. At Crossroads and YES TV, I look at our work of creating daily Christian stories, our online streaming service reaching digital audiences, the stories of hope and wisdom that a religious television station brings into thousands of homes, and the life-giving encouragement on the Crossroads prayer lines, and I realize I need the Holy Spirit more than ever to guide me. I include this illustration of answered prayer not to boast, but to be among the testimony we referred to earlier; I want to be that one who was touched by God, who leaves the crowd to say, "Thank you!"

My own story of inner healing is long and recorded in the book *Faith, Life and Leadership: 8 Canadian Women Tell Their Stories*, but my life reminds me how constant the Holy Spirit can be in our lives. When I was 18, a charismatic revival was making its way through the Mennonite Bible school I attended. Always curious, I naturally had to investigate.

There are several descriptions in the New Testament of how early Christians were filled with the Holy Spirit: John 1:33, John 3:16, John 11:16, Mark 1:8, Acts 1:5, etc.), but by 1977, when I was a young Bible student, getting baptized in the Holy Spirit was called "charismatic revival." Two dormitory deans led me in a prayer to be baptized in the Holy Spirit and then told me to pray in tongues, whatever that might be.

I have a huge portion of my temperament that is introverted and always needs to go away to process things quietly, so as I left that intimate prayer time with others, I journaled alone, away from others. Later I noticed I had written something in my journal that was in a completely foreign language, a language I did not recognize, the language the Bible calls "tongues." Like the gift of healing, tongues, a prayer language, is given at God's discretion.

Life with God is not passive, and neither is the quest for healing. Our longing for good health will deeply affect our spiritual lives, if we let it be so. If we connect our physical life to spiritual practices, we have a constant reminder to stay in relationship with God. The stories of this book encourage us to be in relationship with God.

As David writes in the Psalms, our bodies are *"fearfully and wonderfully made"* (Psalm 139:14). If we truly believe this, we will treat our bodies with a humble reverence that demonstrates an appreciation of their Maker and His craft.

Imagine you had a friend who was a great sculptor, perhaps a modern-day Leonardo da Vinci, and one year, for your birthday, he presented you with his ultimate masterpiece, telling you he made it specifically for you and that it was now yours to keep. How would you treat this precious gift you had been given? Would you place it somewhere by the door where it could easily be scuffed or chipped? Would you let dust and grease build up on its surface?

God has given you a resilient, mind-bogglingly intricate, and beautiful gift. Think about your "friend" who has given you his masterpiece. What would it communicate to him if he came to your house and saw you were treating his work with neglect or even abuse? What an insult! It would mean that you didn't recognize the value of the gift that you had been given, or didn't care about the thought, effort, and time, he had put into it.

To fully grasp the value of what you have been given always leads to humbled awe and thankfulness, and true thankfulness will always affect how we treat both the gift and the giver.

Letting God be God

In the Old Testament story of Job, our protagonist is a man richly blessed in all areas of life. He has a large family of ten children, a bounty of land and livestock, respect and esteem in the community, his health, and a strong faith in the Lord to boot. Yet in a mysterious exchange, Satan complains to God that Job is only faithful because of what God gives him, and that if the things were taken away, Job's true character would be revealed and he would curse God to His face.

God then agrees that Job shall take Satan's proposed test. In two phases of testing, all of Job's children are killed instantly, along with his livestock and servants, and finally Job himself is afflicted with painful sores all over his body. Job responds by tearing his clothes, covering himself in sackcloth and ashes, and crying out to God. But while he does question God, even getting awfully close to accusing God, he never curses Him.

When Job's friends show up, at first, they do the right thing and simply mourn with passionate sympathy alongside Job. But their second course of action isn't as good. One by one, they claim to know the reason behind Job's suffering, and by so confidently knowing the reason, they also claim to know the solution. But Job knows better than his friends. He dismisses their reasoning and goes on directly questioning God. That is, until God quiets the small crowd by showing up Himself. And when He does, He delivers a powerful address that can more or less be summarized by a slight paraphrase of one of His first lines: "I am God, and who are you?"

> Where were you when I laid the earth's foundation?
> Tell me, if you understand.
> Who marked off its dimensions? Surely you know!
> Who stretched a measuring line across it?...
> Have you ever given orders to the morning,
> or shown the dawn its place,
> that it might take the earth by the edges
> and shake the wicked out of it?...
> Have the gates of death been shown to you?
> Have you seen the gates of the deepest darkness?
> Have you comprehended the vast expanses of the earth?
> Tell me, if you know all this...

For Your Health

Have you entered the storehouses of the snow
or seen the storehouses of the hail,
which I reserve for times of trouble,
for days of war and battle?
What is the way to the place where the lightning is
dispersed,
or the place where the east winds are scattered over
the earth?...
Do you hunt the prey for the lioness
and satisfy the hunger of the lions
when they crouch in their dens
or lie in wait in a thicket?
"Does the hawk take flight by your wisdom
and spread its wings toward the south?
Does the eagle soar at your command
and build its nest on high?
"Would you discredit my justice?
Would you condemn me to justify yourself?
Do you have an arm like God's,
and can your voice thunder like his?
Then I myself will admit to you
that your own right hand can save you.

　　　　—JOB 38:4–5, 12–13, 17–18, 22–24,
　　　　　39–40, 39:26–27, 40:8–9, 14

To God's address, Job can only reply:

I know that you can do all things; no purpose of yours
can be thwarted. You asked, "Who is this that ob-
scures my plans without knowledge?" Surely I spoke

114

of things I did not understand, things too wonderful
for me to know.

—JOB 42:2–3

Theologian Timothy Keller notes that such an awe-inspiring monologue may distract us from an interesting fact: God never actually gives Job an answer.[110] For the entire book, Job has been asking God, "Why?" And God never gives Him an answer. Or perhaps He does, and it's just not the kind of answer we would expect. The answer He gives is simply, "I am God, and who are you?"

Those of us living centuries after this book was written may be able to contribute some details to that answer that Job himself never received. In his sermon on Job, Keller asks, is there any other story in literature that is more often referred to as a source of hope in suffering? Can you imagine the number of people [for whom] Job has been a pillar of strength, encouragement, and faith? Certainly Job couldn't have at the time! Even if God gave him some idea, surely his mind wouldn't have been able to comprehend the vastness of the world and the diversity of cultures and time periods that his story would reach.

And so, when Job asked why, we might paraphrase God's brilliantly straightforward response as, "Because I am God and you are you. I've given ample evidence that I am able to do vastly more than you can hope or imagine, and whatever I've done has always been with perfect wisdom, goodness, and might. Let me do my work. Your only job is to trust me."[111]

In the New Testament, we see a somewhat different spin on this same theme. Saul was a highly respected Jewish teacher, chasing down and persecuting that new ragtag bunch of bothersome Christians when Christ met him face-to-face on a highway. As part of this divine encounter, Saul (who would soon become Paul) was afflicted with blindness for three days. But it was partially this temporary blindness that led the way for Paul to see truly for the first time in his life. Saul experienced affliction, but it was not without purpose, or something that had escaped the attention of God. Rather, it was something God used directly for the eternal glory of both Paul and His kingdom.

Romans 8:28 says, *"And we know that in all things God works for the good of those who love him, who have been called according to his purpose."* For some of us who have been in the church for a while, this verse, unfortunately might have become a bit of a cliché. But if it has, stop and truly meditate on it for a while.

In all things, even the ones that seem wicked and broken and horrible, God is working for your good. This good may not be the one you're imagining, it may be a good of the refining, more eternally valuable kind, but it is a good you will look back on one day, a good over which you will worship God in shock and awe and brilliant delight.

FROM THE PRAYER LINES AT CROSSROADS

For Physical Healing:

Heavenly Father, in Jesus' name, we come boldly to Your throne of grace to receive healing for _____ (name of person) from _____ (type of illness). (Hebrews 4:16)

We release Your Word over him/her, believing that Your Word will not return to You empty, but that it will accomplish what You desire, and that it will achieve the purpose for which it is sent. (Isaiah 55:11)

Lord, we agree that Your desire for _____ (name of person) is for him/her to prosper in all things and be in health even as his/her soul prospers. (3 John 2)

We believe that through the sacrifice of Jesus on the cross You provided for _____ (name of person) total healing, and we declare that by the stripes of Jesus, he/she is healed. We pray that _____ (name of person) would experience Your healing touch upon his/her body today. (Isaiah 53:5)

In Jesus' name, we ask that _____ (name of person) would be totally set free from every infirmity, and that Your Spirit that raised Jesus from the dead will raise him/her up (Luke 13:12). We also pray, Father, that any doctor who may be attending to _____ (name of person) will be filled with Your divine wisdom and ability. (Proverbs 4:21–22)

Lord, may Your grace, be poured out upon _____ (name of person) even now. May You help him/her to be strong in faith, keeping Your Word continually within his/her heart and before his/her eyes, for Your Word is life and health to his/her whole body. Thank You, Father, for sending Your Word and healing him/her. (Psalm 107:20)

In faith we declare Your promise of Jeremiah 30:17 over _____ (name of person): *"But I will restore you to health and heal your wounds."* In Jesus' name we pray, Amen. (2 Timothy 1:7)

For Emotional Healing:

Heavenly Father, in Jesus' name, we come boldly to Your throne of grace lifting up _____'s (name of person) emotional needs to You. You know every emotion that he/she has been experiencing, so we come to You as the One who heals the brokenhearted and bind up their wounds. (1 John 1:8)

We set ourselves in agreement with Your Word that You have not given _____ (name of person) a spirit of fear (anxiety, depression, confusion), but a spirit of power and of love and of a sound mind.

So today, we ask, Father, that You would release the power of Your Holy Spirit over _____ (name of person) to bring him/her into sound mental and emotional health. Reveal Your perfect, unconditional love to him/her, we pray, and let Your love become the anchor of his/her soul. (2 Corinthians 10:3–5)

Thank You, Lord Jesus, that You came to destroy the works of the devil; and, in the authority of Your name, we pray that every root of fear, anxiety, worry, confusion, depression, and mental infirmity in _____ (name of person) will be destroyed.

By Your mighty power, we ask You to dissolve the memory and effect of every negative experience that has a hold on his/her mind. Shatter the strongholds, cast down the vain imaginations, and we ask You to give _____ (name of person) the grace to bring every thought into captivity and obedience to Christ. (Hebrews 4:16; Psalm 147:3)

Help _____ (name of person), we pray, not to be anxious about anything, but in everything by prayer and supplication with thanksgiving to make his/her requests known to You, so that Your supernatural peace would guard his/her mind and thoughts through Christ Jesus. We believe, even now, Lord, that You are giving _____ (name of person) the strength to think only on things that are true, noble, just, pure, lovely, praiseworthy, and of good report. Thank You for Your promise, Lord, that You will keep _____ (name of person) in perfect peace as his/her mind is stayed on You. (Philippians 4:6–8)

In faith, we speak Your provision of Isaiah 61:1–3 for _____ (name of person): A crown of beauty instead of ashes, the oil of gladness instead of mourning, and a garment of praise instead of a spirit of despair. In Jesus' name, Amen. (Isaiah 26:3)

These prayers are part of the standard practice resource binder for prayer partners who receive over 1,000 calls each day at Crossroads Christian Communications.

AUTHOR BIOGRAPHIES

Lorna Dueck serves as the CEO of the Crossroads Global Media Group and YES TV network. For over fifteen years, Lorna has been a commentary writer on faith and public life in Canada's leading national newspaper, *The Globe and Mail*, and the executive producer of the Christian news analysis program, "Context."

Lorna completed a Bachelor of Religious Education at Tyndale University College in Toronto and earned a Master of Arts in Evangelism and Leadership from Wheaton College. She has received honorary doctorate degrees from Trinity, Tyndale, and Briercrest universities. Lorna has been honoured with the Queen's Diamond Jubilee Medal for contributions to Canadian society.

Lorna and her husband, Vern, live in Burlington, Ontario, have been married for more than three decades, and delight in the adventures of their grown son and daughter.

Nell DeBoer graduated with a Master of Religion from Wycliffe College, Toronto School of Theology, and completed her Clinical Pastoral Education at Toronto Western Hospital and Toronto General Hospital. She served as chaplain for the Toronto Hospital Ministry of the Christian Reformed Church and was the second woman to be endorsed as a certified chaplain in the Christian Reformed Church of North America. Her work as a chaplain led her to pursue a Doctor of Ministry, for which she wrote her thesis about healing called "Yearning for Wholeness."

Nell was married to her husband, John, for fifty-two years until he passed away in 2013. She lives in Toronto and has five adult children and seventeen grandchildren.

HOW TO GET MORE

All the interviews and stories featured in *For Your Health* are available for you to view online at Crossroads' video streaming platform, Castle™.

These stories have been captured along with scriptural insights and teaching points for viewing with a small group or personal study.

Please visit
www.intothecastle.com/foryourhealth
to request your discount code for full access.

ENDNOTES

1   http://paulteskeministries.com

2   http://robbiedawkins.com

3   Genesis 18:10–14.

4   II Kings 4:16–17.

5   I Kings 17:17–23 and II Kings 4:18–37.

6   II Kings 5:1–14.

7   II Kings 13:21.

8   Michael L. Brown, *Israel's Divine Healer* (Grand Rapids, Michigan: Zondervan, 1995), 167.

9   Morton Kelsey, *Healing & Christianity: A Classical Study,* 3rd ed. (Minneapolis: Augsburg, 1995), 35.

10   Beate Jakob, "The Human Being is a Multidimensional Unity," Neglected Dimensions in Health and Healing (Tubingen: German Institute for Medical Mission, 2001), 29.

11   Jakob, 29, Luke 11:20.

12   Jakob, 29.

13   Jakob, 29.

14   Acts 2.

15   Acts 3.

16   John Wilkinson, *The Bible and Healing* (Grand Rapids, Michigan: Eerdmans, 1998), Chapter 15.

17   II Corinthians 12.

18   Philippians 2.

19   I Timothy 5:23.

20   II Timothy 4:11.

21   Wilkinson, 193.

22   Evelyn Frost, *Christian Healing*. (Lond: A.R. Mowbray, 1949), 17.

23   Frost, 70.

24   Cited in Frost, 64.

25   Frost, 64.

26   Frost, 103.

27   Frost, 99.

28   Frost, 64–5 and 104–5.

29   Frost, 67–8 and 104–6.

30   Frost, 67–8 and 104–6.

31   Frost, 68, 43, 46, and 107.

32   Kelsey, 126.

33   Kelsey, 126.

34   Citing Saint Augustine, City of God, XXII.8, in Kelsey, 145–6.

35   Kelsey, 151–2.

36   Kelsey, 151–2.

37   Jakob, 31–32.

38   Henry Wildeboer, *Miraculous Healing and You* (Grand Rapids: CRC Publications, 1999), 56.

39   Kelsey, 17.

40   Kelsey, 17.

41   Kelsey, 17.

42   Jon Ruthven, *On the Cessation of the Charismata: The Protestant Polemic on Postbiblical Miracles*. (Sheffield, England: Sheffield Academic Press, 1993), 34.

43 Calvin, Institutes, IV.XIX.18.

44 Calvin, Institutes, IV.XIX.19.

45 Ruthven, 197-200.

46 Gary B. McGee, "Mission, the Divine/Human Enterprise," *International Bulletin of Missionary Research*, 25, no. 4 (October 2001).

47 Stanley M. Burgess, Gary B. McGee, Ed., and Patrick H. Alexander, Assoc. Ed., "The Gift of Healing" in Dictionary of Pentecostal & Charismatic Movements, 1989, 353.

48 Burgess, 353–354.

49 Donald W. Dayton, *Theological Roots of Pentecostalism.* (Metuchen, NJ: Scarecrow, 1987), 118–119.

50 Burgess, 361.

51 Andrew Murray, *Divine Healing* (New Kensington, PA: Whitaker House, 1982), 5.

52 Murray, 5.

53 Murray, 24–25.

54 Burgess, 373.

55 Dayton, 117.

56 Francis MacNutt, "Healing by Everyone," Sharing Magazine, August 2001, 5–10.

57 Wildeboer, 92.

58 James 5:13–16.

59 Acts of Synod, 1973, 453–4.

60 Elisabeth Elliot, *Facing the Death of Someone You Love* (Wheaton, Illinois: Crossway, 2012), 7.

61 Elliot, 7.

62 Elliot, 7.

63 Elliot, 9.

64 Elliot, 9.

65 David B. Larson, Spirituality and Medical Outcomes: A Presentation at the Spirituality & Healing in Medicine Conference (Chicago, March 20, 1999).

66 Harold G. Koenig, *The Healing Power of Faith: Science Explores Medicine's Last Great Frontier* (New York: Simon & Schuster, 1999), 12.

67 Koenig, 20–21.

68 Koenig, 33.

69 Koenig, 24.

70 Dale A. Matthews, *The Faith Factor: Proof of the Healing Power of Prayer* (New York: Viking, 1998), 2–3.

71 Matthews, 2.

72 Matthews, 18

73 Matthews, 16.

74 Matthews, 18.

75 Christoph Benn, "Does Faith Contribute to Healing?" Neglected Dimensions in Health and Healing, Study Document No. 3. (Tubingen, Germany: German Institute for Medical Mission, 2001), 49.

76 Jeff Levin, Ph.D. *God, Faith, and Health: Exploring the Spirituality-Healing Connection* (New York: J. Wiley, 2001), 41.

77 Levin, 41.

78 Levin, 57–66.

79 Levin, 81.

80 Levin, 89.

81 Levin, 90.

82 Levin, 91.

83 Levin, 98–99.

84 Levin, 129.

85 Levin, 138

86 Levin, 146.

87   Levin, 151.

88   Levin, 155.

89   Levin, 163.

90   Levin, 156.

91   Levin, 161.

92   Levin, 177.

93   Levin, 159.

94   Levin, 199–201.

95   Howard L. Rice, *Reformed Spirituality* (Louisville: Westminster/John Knox, 1991), 71.

96   Rice, 74.

97   Rice, 83–85.

98   Rice, 82–83.

99   Citing Randolph Byrd, "Positive Therapeutic Effects of Intercessory Prayer in a Coronary Care Unit Population," Southern Medical Journal 81 (1988), 826–29., in Matthews, 199–200.

100 Barbara Fiand, *Prayer and the Quest for Healing* (New York: Crossroad Publishing Company, 2000), 151.

101 Fiand, 151.

102 John Polkinghorne, Larry Dossey, and Herbert Benson, *Healing Through Prayer* (Toronto: Dundurn Press, 2002), 21.

103 Polkinghorne, 22.

104 Larry Dossey, *Healing Words: The Power of Prayer and the Practice of Medicine* (San Francisco: Harper, 1993), xv.

105 Dossey, xviii.

106 Polkinghorne, 35.

107 Ronald Rolheiser, *The Holy Longing: The Search for a Christian Spirituality* (New York: Doubleday, 1999), 53 and 66.

108 Richard Foster, *The Celebration of Discipline* (San Francisco: Harper, 1998).

109 Polkinghorne, 16.

110 Timothy Keller, "Questions of Suffering." Job: A path through suffering, January 6, 2008, Redeemer Presbyterian, New York City: NY. Sermon.

111 Keller, 2008.